Menopause!
RESET!

Menopause!
RESET!

REVERSE WEIGHT GAIN,
SPEED FAT LOSS,
AND GET YOUR BODY BACK
IN 3 SIMPLE STEPS

MICKEY HARPAZ, PhD,
with Robert Wolff

RODALE

© 2011 by Mickey Harpaz and Robert Wolff

Rodale books may be purchased for business or promotional use or for special sales. For information, please write to:
Special Markets Department, Rodale Inc., 733 Third Avenue, New York, NY 10017

Printed in the United States of America
Rodale Inc. makes every effort to use acid-free ∞, recycled paper ♺.

The content on pages 165 to 177 of Bonus Section 2 have been reprinted courtesy of the US Food and Drug Administration, November 2004,
http://www.fda.gov/food/labelingnutrition/consumerinformation/ucm078889.htm

Illustrations by Scott Russo
Book design by Rachel Reiss

Library of Congress Cataloging-in-Publication Data

Harpaz, Mickey.
    Menopause reset! : reverse weight gain, speed fat loss, and get your body back in 3 simple steps / Mickey Harpaz, with Robert Wolff.
        p.   cm.
    ISBN–13 978–1–60961–447–8   paperback
    1. Menopause—Popular works.   2. Women—Diseases—Diet therapy.
I. Wolff, Robert.   II. Title.
RG186.H37   2010
618.1'75—dc22   2010026539

Distributed to the trade by Macmillan
2   4   6   8   10   9   7   5   3   1   paperback

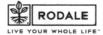

We inspire and enable people to improve their lives and the world around them.
rodalebooks.com

To the three women in my life—

I dedicate this book in loving memory to my grandmother Saftona, my role model and best friend. She was a gentle woman who walked the earth in peace and kindness, teaching my family and me how to find happiness and be happy each and every day.

To my loving mother, Pnina, a strong woman whose actions throughout all of her life, taught me the vast power of perseverance, dedication, and family values.

To my partner, Ingrid, whose love and support will forever bring warmth to the meaning of my life. I am immeasurably indebted to you, Ingrid, for your intelligence and insight, patience and compassion, which are everything I could ask for.

Contents

Preface

It was a beautiful spring day outside my office. Inside, the scene was a little gloomier.

Barbara was sitting in my office waiting for me to come in.

I walked in and smiled and said, "Hello, Barbara, and how are—"

"If this continues," she interrupted with a look of frustration, "I will have to live on the treadmill for hours each day just so I won't get any fatter!"

I knew she was joking, but I also knew that Barbara's lament wasn't that far from the truth.

You see, Barbara was on a journey that millions of women like her are on, a journey called *menopause* that leaves many scared, unsure, and in emotional tatters as they try to figure out what is happening inside their bodies and how long the uncertainty and physical and emotional challenges will go on.

Barbara then asked a question that I have always remembered.

"Dr. Harpaz," she began, "why is it that the older I become, the more I exercise, and the less I eat, the *fatter* I am?

"And why is it that I've gained so much weight—a weight I previously would have associated with the second trimester of pregnancy or perhaps having a daily midmorning glazed doughnut and a candy bar—despite my daily 2 hours of a grueling yoga class followed by a workout at the gym?"

She continued, "I'm still not sure how midlife weight gain managed to sneak up on me in my forties. It's not as if I ignored all the troubling public health bulletins about the snowball effects of overeating. I know that women's bodies gradually burn fewer calories because of the declining estrogen levels."

Barbara, like so many women her age, was frustrated, unmotivated, annoyed, and sometimes even livid about the midlife weight gain that had snuck up on her.

In this Twitter age of instant information (and of the plethora of it that's out there, much of it is confusing), it's not as if women ignore the media coverage and all the news about the snowball effects of aging.

What many women *don't* realize is the *importance* and *consequences* of their bodies gradually burning fewer calories over time and of the ever-decreasing estrogen levels that cause fat to be deposited where beautiful and shapely muscle once was.

And they have very similar reactions and responses.

Barbara explained it well.

"After a month of religiously adhering to a grueling exercise program and reducing my caloric intake to minuscule amounts, my success was measured as a pathetic 1-pound loss on the scale. And my aggravation level went sky-high! I looked in a mirror, pointed a finger at my double-crossing body, and declared all-out war. 'You are going to lose weight or else!' I am at my wit's end! I don't know what else I can do."

At that point Barbara looked at me and in a desperate, exasperated voice she whispered, "Help!"

Sound familiar?

It does to me because I see it all the time. I've seen it in the more than 10,000 women I've helped during my more than 20 years in practice.

You see, Barbara could just as easily be any woman.

Yes, even you.

And if you've ever felt helpless, powerless, and frustrated in the face of something you've believed was out of your control, then I've got good news.

Menopause Reset! will give you the direction, diet recommendations, and physiological strategies to reverse the menopause weight gain you've been experiencing.

Just like they did for Barbara. This is what I told her:

"Barbara," I answered, "we can tackle this obstacle together and succeed.

"I can provide direction and physiological strategies to *reverse* the menopause weight gain process. So are you ready to face the challenge?"

She smiled, nodded, and for the first time during the appointment she appeared to relax and look hopeful.

"However," I continued, "the necessary ingredients for weight control success for menopausal women like you are, first, an understanding of a woman's physiology and what happens during menopause. Second, I need for you to follow my guidelines. Third, and perhaps most important, do you have a deep desire and are you motivated to succeed?"

With a big smile, Barbara nodded her head to indicate an enthusiastic *yes*! She was ready.

And with *Menopause Reset!* so are you!

Introduction

Menopause can be a devastating and debilitating state that wreaks physical and emotional havoc on the lives of the women going through it.

Forty-five million women in *just* the United States are menopausal right now. Each day, thousands of women join their numbers. With its typical effects, including hot flashes, fatigue, hair loss, bloating, allergies, mood swings, depression, anxiety, migraines, digestive problems, irritability, panic disorder, joint pain, breast pain, whole body discomfort, osteoporosis, and more, menopausal women need help they haven't been able to find.

Until now.

Welcome to *Menopause Reset!*

A Doctor, a Program, and a Book Whose Time Has Come

Until now, menopausal women have lived without the help of a definitive plan that would ameliorate their symptoms and give them the solutions they seek, especially for weight and fat loss.

The problem is, they've been following diets and exercise plans directed at women of any age.

Only after months, years, and many thousands of dollars do menopausal women find out the harsh reality: The diets and exercise programs they've been following simply don't work because they aren't designed to attack and eliminate the causes and symptoms of weight and fat gain that are specific to menopause.

In fact, in the October 2008 issue of the *Journal of Obesity*, David Yankura, MD, of the University of Pittsburgh School of Medicine, and his colleagues reported that 95 percent of menopausal women who diet will regain as much as *two-thirds* of the weight they lose within 1 year of completing a diet program, and almost all of it within 5 years.

Only *3 percent* of those who take off the weight will keep it off for at least 5 years.

Nine out of 10 American premenopausal and menopausal women will gain weight (as will 70 percent of all women worldwide, due to varied diets and other cultural influences), says Amos Pines, MD, former president of the International Menopause Society. They can expect to gain 10 to 20 pounds, which translates into needing clothing that's one or two sizes larger. Many menopausal women become frustrated, discouraged, annoyed, and even livid as they gain the weight.

Far too often, the menopausal woman's reaction to such a dramatic weight gain is to resort to a drastic starvation diet to rid herself of the extra pounds.

Rarely does it work.

Each time a menopausal woman tries a diet of deprivation, the weight becomes more difficult to lose due to physiological changes these diets cause, making her even more discouraged, which often results in overeating and triggers a cascade of new and unwanted side effects.

With all this frustration and lack of success in reaching weight and fat loss goals, the menopausal woman's mind-set goes from one of healthy, strong self-esteem to self-doubt and lack of confidence in her ability to change. She may give up and accept what she thinks is a new reality: She is destined to be overweight.

I KNOW YOU ARE READY

The big question is, With tens of millions of women experiencing menopause right now, why is it that no diet program has been able to give them the help they need?

The answer: Because no one has understood how food, diet, and exercise affect the menopausal woman. But now, a doctor who has found out what *works* has developed the perfect program for menopausal women—one that has been designed *just* for them.

It's a plan designed specifically to lessen their symptoms, change their bodies, and *reverse* the negative effects of menopausal weight and fat gain.

With *Menopause Reset!* menopausal women will no longer need to ask, "Why is it that the older I become, the more I exercise, and the less I eat, the fatter I get?"

And for any menopausal woman who has ever felt powerless and cried out, "I want my body back!" there's good news.

She's about to get it.

It's taken 20 years and more than 10,000 women, but now it's time for menopausal women worldwide to meet the doctor who devised this revolutionary program that's about to dramatically change their lives for the better.

It's time for *Menopause Reset!*

What to Expect from *Menopause Reset!*

The power of *Menopause Reset!* has been proven with the results of more than 10,000 women—women just like you—through more than 20 years of use.

The real-world results of real people are powerful testimonials to the benefits that *Menopause Reset!* will bring. Benefits that you can expect to experience include:

PHYSIOLOGICAL AND PSYCHOLOGICAL CHANGES AND BENEFITS

- Higher energy levels and lower fatigue levels

- Increased productivity in all facets of daily life

- Better-quality sleep

- Increased mood stability

- Decreased stress level

- Decreased depression level

- Increased self-esteem

WEIGHT LOSS AND FAT LOSS CHANGES AND BENEFITS

- Stopped and reversed menopausal weight gain

- Fat loss at a rate of 0.5 percent of total body fat *per week*

- Weight loss at a rate of 0.5 to 1.25 pounds *per week*

- Dropping *two or three* clothing sizes within the 1st year on the program

And this is only the beginning.

We're about to change your menopausal body and life in ways no one has told you about.

It's time for you to take control of menopause and get your body back. Turn the page and *Menopause Reset!* will show you how.

Menopause!
RESET!

CHAPTER 1

How *Menopause Reset!* Came to Be

When I was studying for my doctorates in applied physiology and nutrition from Columbia and Belford universities, I became very interested in how certain factors affect human weight gain and loss.

I studied nearly every diet that had been popular over the previous 30 years, and I was curious about why some diets worked for some people, but not as well for others. And about why the same diet may produce better results in a woman than in a man, and vice versa.

As I began collecting data from my dietary research, I became interested in the weight gain and weight loss problems of menopause-age women that I was hearing about and observing firsthand. I wanted to know why the diets that worked for younger women were not working with equal success (or at all) for menopausal women.

And, I noticed, there weren't any effective diet books (based on peer-reviewed science) that specifically focused on the menopausal woman.

LET THE EXPERIMENTATION BEGIN

In the late 1980s, I began shifting my practice and its focus to helping women—specifically, menopausal women—diminish the severity of the unwanted side effects of menopause. The goal was to help them achieve sustainable weight and fat loss and improve their overall health. In other words, to give them their bodies back.

The first area I focused on was diet.

I experimented with every kind of popular diet that was available, and the results were less than spectacular. So I created my own. And for my menopausal patients, the results were (and continue to be) stunning.

Then I took on exercise.

I looked at the decades-old traditional methods of training (and hundreds of workouts that ranged from using weights to running to doing cardio and other modalities) and began applying them in numerous variations in the lives of my menopausal patients. Years of observation and empirical research helped me create and fine-tune the ideal exercise regimen that the menopausal woman's body needs and will respond best to.

And finally, there was the mental aspect.

One of the big mistakes I felt so many diet and exercise books made was either neglecting or totally disregarding the importance of the brain and how it affects how we think and feel. We are a brain with a body and not the other way around. And the unchangeable truth is, where the mind goes, the body follows.

And I discovered something even more astounding: The mind greatly affects menopausal weight and fat gain and loss. The connection is huge.

Once I knew all of this, identifying my goal was simple: Bring the mind, the diet, and the exercise regimen together so they would work in perfect harmony in the menopausal woman's body and create something I call the reset.

Reset *thinking*. Reset *diet*. Reset *movement*.

To start the reset and keep it going, there are three steps: the mental reset, the diet reset, and the physical reset. By themselves, none has the power to push a menopausal woman's reset button. But if you use all three at the same time (as you will with *Menopause Reset!*), you'll press the reset button—and keep it pressed for a lifetime of great results.

You are about to learn what's taken me more than 20 years and 10,000 patients to create, fine-tune, and perfect.

For years, millions of menopausal women have been ready for this program, and since you're reading this book, I know that you are, too.

It is time for *Menopause Reset!* to help you.

Throw All the Old Diets Out the Window

My goal in writing this book is to give you the knowledge and power to make great lifestyle choices and changes that will positively affect your health, conditioning, and general well-being.

As an exercise physiologist and nutritionist, I'm a specialist in helping people change their lifestyles so the bodies they have are the bodies they want.

Bodies that are healthy, strong, vibrant, and energetic.

Bodies that they can spend the rest of their lives enjoying.

We will improve your health and well-being by enhancing your body's ability to metabolize food, strengthening its immune system, and increasing your energy level—all at the same time.

And here's some good news: You will do all of it—and lose weight—*without feeling deprived or hungry.* Armed with the information you are about to learn and the motivation to follow the plan, as my thousands of patients will attest, you will *never* fall into the trap of dieting again!

So let's talk about the word *diet.*

I want you to think of the word *diet* as a reference to a way of life. That's all.

Diet in this book refers to the way you eat as part of your lifestyle. It is behavior patterns. It is eating the right foods in the proper amounts and at the correct times of the day. In this book, *diet* does *not* refer to a restricted caloric intake program that you employ to lose weight.

By following the *Menopause Reset!* principles, you will:

- Build and maintain a vital metabolism

- Increase your daily activity and exercise levels

- Learn the core proper eating habits

- Integrate the latest nutritional facts into a commonsense eating approach that will increase your energy and improve your overall health

- Regulate your blood glucose and insulin levels to burn fat

SO MANY HEADLINES—HOW CAN YOU KNOW WHAT'S TRUE?

Not a day passes without a new finding about food and its effect on us being publicized. We are bombarded with so much news about food, exercise, and health. So why is it, despite all of this information that's instantly available to us, so many of us keep getting fatter every day?

A big reason: *Conventional diets do not work!*

This is especially true for menopausal women. The menopausal body is an intricate physiological machine with a different set of rules and regulations.

By the time you finish this book, you will have a good working understanding of nutrition and physiology, and this powerful knowledge will give you *all* of the tools you need to take control of your body and avoid falling victim to the diet trap again.

If you look in the dictionary, you'll find that the primary definition of *diet* refers to the sort of food a person typically eats. A secondary definition narrows that to the foods a person is limited to eating for medical reasons. Note that there's no mention of calorie or nutrient restriction or deprivation, or of hunger.

So from this point on, let's think of the word *diet* as simply your way of eating, with good eating habits, the foods that supply you with the proper nutrition. That's all.

You may be asking, "Is it really possible to learn the right kind of diet habits that will last me a lifetime?"

I'll let Tina, one of my clients, give you the answer.

> *I joined your program and within 8 weeks had not only made*
> *major impacts in weight and general conditioning, but also*
> *experienced direct health benefits with respect to a lung condition*
> *and an operation-affected muscle area.*
>
> *By learning about food and its roles in my life from the*
> *nutritional and physiological standpoints, I was able to change*
> *and realign my old eating habits. More importantly, I could*
> *easily make this adjustment, and with a positive attitude.*

Along with the positive diet changes you'll enjoy making, the exercise changes will be seamless and fit into your life like a glove.

And it all begins with your mind and perceptions.

When Paula, a former county attorney, came into my office, she knew exactly what she wanted.

> *I want my energy level back. I only need to lose 15 pounds, but*
> *more importantly, I'd like to tone my muscles and lose my fat. I*
> *need to reduce my borderline high blood pressure, and I believe*
> *that as I reach these goals, my resting blood pressure will return*
> *to normal. However, I have one condition that I insist upon: No*
> *one, but no one, will take my evening dry martini away from me.*

Let me tell you, Paula kept her evening dry martini, closed an old chapter in her lifestyle, reached her goals, got her body and energy back, and never dieted again.

Janet came to my office 35 pounds overweight and suffering from chronic fatigue syndrome. This debilitating condition had forced her to quit her job and drained her of energy and hope. That day, Janet began a life-changing transition to new eating and exercise habits based on the *Menopause Reset!* regimen outlined in this book. She has never turned back.

I met Roberta, the dean of a graduate school, at the health club where she worked out. Ready to make some changes in her life after the New Year's holiday, she came to my office and related a medical history that included stress from a high-pressure job, menopause overweight, high blood pressure, high cholesterol, and very poor eating habits. Overwhelmed by her situation, Roberta knew she had to augment her doctorate-level education with some straight, hard facts on nutrition.

> *I want my body and energy back. I cannot afford to continue like this. I need to lose weight and I must eat better, not to mention reduce my blood pressure.*
>
> *The stress and the pressure at work do not help. I need a good exercise program to relieve those.*

Since that day, my well-educated dean has earned high marks in successfully implementing the *Menopause Reset!* program, and she's never looked back.

Since 1987, I have treated more than 10,000 clients like Tina, Paula, Janet, and Roberta. Each came to me desperately needing to lose her menopausal weight gain, stop the yo-yo dieting syndrome, or improve a wide variety of health conditions. And each graduated from my program with priceless degrees in proper nutrition and exercise.

You, my friend, will do the same.

CHAPTER 2

Why Diet Plans Don't Work (and *Menopause Reset!* Does)

If you've been frustrated and discouraged by all the years of failed diets, weight gain, weight loss, and weight gain again or are confused and at a loss to know what to do or who and what you should trust, you are in good company.

We are a nation of diet-obsessed people, and there are countless programs, pills, and people out there dispensing different messages about how to take weight off.

About one-half of American women and one-fourth of American men are currently trying to lose weight, and another one-fourth in each gender group are trying to maintain their current weight. One out of three females between the ages of 11 and 18 is on a diet plan to lose weight.

To make matters even more confusing, weight gradually creeps up on us as we age. Between the ages of 20 and 45, we add an average of 1 to 2 pounds a year. The fact that we are overweight may not hit us until one day when we wake up and find that we're carrying around 20 to 60 pounds of excess fat. We realize that we don't look good and don't feel good, and that the excess fat is likely to shorten our lives. So, we resolve to go on a diet plan.

7

Between the ages of 20 and 45, Americans collectively lose millions of pounds on various diet plans. During this period of time each of us belongs to an average of 17 health clubs, and many visit diet institutes and spas and go on weight loss getaways, all while starting seemingly endless numbers of diet programs.

Yes, we may successfully lose weight, but the weight *inevitably* comes back, and in many instances we *surpass* the weight we were at before we started that great new diet plan.

WHY *NOT* DIET?

Let me ask you a question: If diets do not work for the general population, why would anyone think they would work for the menopausal woman?

Consider the following 1998 statistic (the most current comprehensive survey data available): Since 1920, there have been 28,000 diet plans published in the United States. Twenty-eight thousand different types of diets! The American Heart Association published the results of a survey indicating that 95 to 98 percent of people starting a new diet plan will regain the weight within the first 2 to 5 years and in many cases will gain even more weight than they lost.

A similar study indicates that the American diet industry had sales of $29 billion in 1998 alone. The following year, the figure increased to $31 billion. Moreover, the study found that $30 billion of the $31 billion in the second year was spent by the same people who spent the $29 billion the previous year!

YOU SIMPLY CANNOT WIN AT WEIGHT LOSS BY DIETING

It is physiologically impossible to lose 3 pounds of fat, not water, from the body in 1 week, much less the 5-pound drop that some commercial diet plans advertise that they can deliver.

If only 1 percent of the published diets delivered what they promise, we would all be slim and trim by now and you would not be reading this book.

And if diet plans work, then why are we fatter than ever?

And why are our children 100 percent fatter than we were when we were children in the 1970s?

IT'S TIME FOR A REALITY CHECK

We must be honest with ourselves.

Look around at the mall, in the supermarket, at work. Look at our friends, our families, and the strangers in the streets. What do you see?

We are fat!

There is enough fat on enough of us to feed one-third of the human race.

Think about that.

It should be obvious that with scores of new diet plans being published every year, each one claiming to be just what you need, something fishy is going on.

Year after year, fad diets come and go and yet we always get suckered into following them—even though we know that a fad diet is just that. It will not change our eating behaviors and habits, and it will not result in sustainable weight loss.

Americans are currently eating fewer calories than we did in 1900, yet more of us are overweight than ever before.

How can this be? According to research published in the journal *Nutrition Research* in 2009, traditional diets may cause a wide variety of health problems.

Dieting is correlated with a strong tendency to regain weight, with as much as two-thirds of the weight lost being regained within 1 year of completing a program—and almost *all* of it within 5 years.

Think about how many of us try to lose weight by counting calories, carefully keeping track of everything we consume, and depriving ourselves by limiting the amount of food we eat.

And if you've ever tried the packaged diet foods, you've probably discovered just how unappealing they are. It takes only a short time of counting every calorie and eating foods you dislike for you to quickly grow tired of all the trouble and hunger in your life. And then it happens: You abandon the diet plan and regain the weight you lost, and sometimes, you put on even more.

In a review article published in the journal *Archives of Internal Medicine*, Kelly Brownell, PhD, and Judith Rodin, PhD, of Yale University found that only about 3 percent of those who take off weight keep it off for at least 5 years. Worse than this is that the yo-yo syndrome of dieting—losing some weight, then gaining it back—may be more harmful to your health than staying a little heavy.

It's time for us to break the pattern and put an end to this frustrating behavior once and for all.

WHAT TRADITIONAL DIET PLANS HAVE PROVEN TO DELIVER

So you might be asking, "Well, Dr. Harpaz, aren't there any things that diet plans *do* do?" Glad you asked! But the answers may not be what you expect.

- **DEVELOP UNCONSCIOUS EATING HABITS.** Letting someone else dictate when and what you should eat rather than listening to your body and understanding when you're full or hungry can encourage mindless eating—not a good habit to get into. I'd rather be conscious when I decide what to put in my mouth.

- **BRING UP FEELINGS OF DEPRIVATION.** It's a dangerous myth that you have to feel deprived in order to lose weight. In fact, the research shows that deprivation can actually lead to weight gain. *It is scandalous to feel deprived in this food-rich country.*

- **CREATE STRESS.** Stress has been linked conclusively to weight gain. Don't you already have enough stress in your life? Daily commuting stress is enough for me.

- **CAUSE BOREDOM.** Conventional diet plans tend to encourage you to stick to one food group over all others. With more than 10,000 food items in supermarkets, you can find lots of fun food choices and meal combinations. Why be bored?

- **ENCOURAGE MEAL SKIPPING.** Skipping meals can have a negative effect on your metabolism. If you need to skip anything, skip rope, not meals.

- **FEED LOW SELF-ESTEEM AND A LACK OF SELF-TRUST AND FAITH.** Don't let the diet purveyors blame you for their lack of success in helping you lose weight. Stop participating in those diets, and start building your faith in yourself and what you are doing.

- **CAUSE EXCESSIVE HUNGER.** Allowing hunger to take over encourages overeating. *Menopause Reset!* will teach you how to eat six or more small meals a day. You'll be happier, and excessive hunger will be a thing of the past.

- **PROVOKE UNREALISTIC EXPECTATIONS.** Losing 40 pounds in 40 days has never happened healthfully for anyone! Be honest with yourself and your dreams will become reality.

- **SAP STRENGTH, MOTIVATION, ENERGY, AND MUSCLE.** Once you realize the old way of dieting doesn't work, you'll be ready for *Menopause Reset!* It's time for you to look and feel fantastic.

LOW CALORIES AND FASTING ARE BIG NO-NOS

Let's talk a little bit more about low caloric diet plans and fasting.

A review article published recently in the *International Journal of Sport Nutrition and Exercise Metabolism* revealed that low-calorie diets and fasting are associated with a variety of short-term adverse effects, including fatigue, hair loss, and dizziness. More serious was that the risk of developing gallstones and acute gallbladder disease increased during severe caloric restriction.

Then there are those diet plans that may cause medical problems by telling you to eat particular foods or kinds of foods. This is especially true of the high-protein plans that recommend that you increase your consumption of meats and eggs and reduce your carbohydrate intake. This can increase the risk of heart disease, stroke, kidney disease, and many other health problems. And for those who experience rapid weight loss on these diets, the reality is that the lost weight—primarily water—is just as rapidly regained.

Aside from the health risks, the fact is that when you go on a diet plan of deprivation, weight becomes more difficult to lose. As a result, dieters tend to become discouraged. This despondency often leads to eating even more, causing more depression, and then more overeating. It's a vicious cycle. Eventually, you blame yourself for being destined to be fat, overweight, or obese, and for lacking willpower—which, in turn, lowers your self-esteem.

What you've been missing is scientifically based information that will enable you to make better choices about your eating habits and your lifestyle. And here's the key: For any weight loss to be successful and to stick, you must make these changes yourself. *Menopause Reset!* will show you how to make slight changes in your lifestyle to make it an active one with the smart and efficient eating habits that are the keys to success.

A PLAN CREATED WITH *YOU* IN MIND

Early on, I discovered just how ineffective diet plans are for the menopausal woman.

You see, three very important key objectives to help the menopausal woman get her body back are to reset her metabolic rate, increase her daily metabolic rate (or DMR, the average rate over the course of a day), and enhance her fat utilization. However, being on a low-calorie diet plan is metabolically counterproductive to all of those goals because it can trigger the following physiological mechanisms:

- Dieting puts the menopausal woman's body in starvation mode, which decreases her DMR.

- Dieting either slows or shuts down the benefit gained from the thermogenic effect of food. (Basically, it takes energy to ingest and digest. In other words, eating burns calories! You will find more about this in the chapter entitled Step 2: Reset Your Diet!)

- Dieting hampers the ability to increase lean body mass, which negatively affects the DMR and caloric output. Moreover, far too many menopausal women dieters do not exercise, and therefore they lose out on exercise's positive metabolic benefit entirely.

The problem is that diet plans, especially for menopausal women, do not attack the fundamental problems (the physiological trigger mechanisms and results listed above). And as ironic as it may seem, at the beginning of a diet cycle, losing weight is clearly not the problem for the overweight person. In fact, most overweight people could make a profession out of losing weight.

Some of us consume amounts of food that healthy-weight people might have a hard time digesting.

Some eat less than nondieters without losing weight.

Some gain weight.

And many used to lose weight, but not anymore.

Now, nothing works.

This strange phenomenon of *eating less yet gaining more* raises many questions.

- Why is it that my friend can easily lose weight and I cannot?

- Why is it that my spouse can eat twice as much as I eat and never gain?

- Why is it that even when I starve myself, I don't lose weight?

- Why is it that as soon as I go on a diet, I am totally starving and cannot stop thinking about food?

SCIENCE GIVES US THE ANSWERS

Scientific research has begun to uncover the physiological bases of these problems. Certain changes that occur in the body on a low-calorie diet and with a low-activity lifestyle make it progressively harder to lose weight and to keep it off. It is not simply a question of

having too-high caloric intake or inadequate output, following a specific diet plan, or having too little willpower.

By going on a diet plan, you actually make it *harder* for your body
to lose weight.

Janet, Tina, Paula, and many more of my patients all faced the
same problem prior to their introduction to *Menopause Reset!* They
had low, sluggish metabolisms.

What is the difference between the hungry slim person and the
hungry fat person? The difference is that one eats and the other fights
it. Usually, it's the thin person who eats.

Then why isn't the thin one fat?

Research published in the *American Journal of Clinical Nutrition* in
2009 found that in order to fire up metabolism and the fat-burning
process, you must take in the proper nutrients and engage in activity.
The last thing you want to do when you have a low metabolism is
restrict your energy input with a low-calorie diet.

This seems counterintuitive to many people who believe that
weight loss requires starvation and restriction. My patient Janet has
struggled with the negative effects of this mentality for her entire
adult life. It started with aerobics and various weight loss programs
when she was in her midtwenties. She just wanted to lose a few
pounds she'd put on during her first years of college.

A commercial diet plan helped her lose a few pounds very quickly,
and she soon looked great and was ready for swimsuit season. However, the plan failed to tell Janet that because it was a low-calorie diet,
it would slow down her metabolism.

Two years later, after graduating from college, Janet found herself
writing a check to a second diet service. This time, she tried a starvation diet—less than 1,000 calories per day.

Once again she lost weight and was ready for the beach. Yet once
again, because of the physiological effects of most diet plans, her
metabolism became even more sluggish.

When I met Janet, she had just given up on the $800 she had
invested in a third weight loss program. She was without hope. Thirty
years after her initial diet (yes, 30 years!) and postmenopausal, she
was 35 pounds overweight, had no muscle tone, and carried a very
high percentage of body fat. Janet had no energy and suffered from
chronic fatigue syndrome. Her metabolism had nearly shut down.

Just Get Started

Use the power of momentum. The hardest thing for many people is getting started, especially when it comes to exercise and eating better. One of the laws of physics states that an object will stay at rest until it's acted upon by an outside force. Let's change that to say: *A body will stay out of shape and lethargic until it's set into action by an inside force.*

That means changing those self-limiting thoughts and beliefs and taking action. Do just a *little* something each day to make your body stronger and healthier. Just one little action, that's all. This sets in motion the power of momentum, and make no mistake, momentum is awesomely powerful.

If you were to place a couple of two-by-fours under the wheels of a 60-ton locomotive, you'd keep it from moving. But once you remove those blocks and let that train start moving and gaining momentum, it will crash through a wall of concrete 10 feet thick! That's the power of momentum, and it's time you use that very same power to change your body and life.

It wasn't until she started on the *Menopause Reset!* program that she began to see the results she'd been working so hard (and fruitlessly) for all those years.

MENOPAUSE: WHAT IT IS

As if the body's response to dieting weren't hard enough to understand, menopause makes matters even more complex.

So what is menopause, exactly? Menopause is the permanent end of menstruation and fertility. It is the date on which a woman hasn't had a menstrual period for a year. Perimenopause is the period of hormonal fluctuation that *leads up to* menopause, and it can last from 5 to 15 years or longer.

And every woman's symptoms are different.

Common symptoms include hot flashes, night sweats, insomnia, irregular periods, loss of libido, and vaginal dryness.

Other changes women may notice are fatigue, hair loss, sleep disorders besides insomnia, difficulty concentrating, memory lapses, dizziness, incontinence, bloating, new allergies, brittle nails, changes in body odor, irregular heartbeat, mood swings, depression, anxiety, irritability, and panic disorder.

Discomfort may be felt bodywide and can include breast pain, migraines, joint pain, a burning sensation on the tongue, electric shock sensations, digestive problems, gum problems, muscle tension, and itchy skin or tingling extremities. Osteoporosis also can begin during this time.

THE HORMONAL TRIGGERS

Weight gain during menopause is the most common symptom for the majority of the female population reaching this stage of their lives. And this is due to changes in the hormone balance that affects weight control, resulting in a condition that I call P-E-A-T.

Progesterone decreases.

Estrogen decreases.

Androgen increases.

Testosterone decreases.

Each of those hormonal components affects the way the menopausal woman's body functions and uses calories.

PROGESTERONE: During menopause, progesterone levels decrease. Lower levels of progesterone can be responsible for menopausal symptoms, including weight gain. Water weight and bloating are also caused by decreased progesterone levels, but those symptoms are not necessarily related to weight gain. They can make clothes feel tight, however, making you *feel* heavier.

ESTROGEN: During a woman's fertile phase of life, estrogen is the female sex hormone responsible for causing monthly ovulation. During menopause, estrogen declines rapidly, causing ovulation to stop.

Estrogen also seems to play a major part in weight gain during menopause. As the menopausal woman's ovaries produce less estrogen, her body looks for other estrogen sources in her body. Fat cells can produce estrogen, so your body works harder to turn calories into fat to increase estrogen levels. Unfortunately for you, fat cells don't burn calories the way muscle cells do, and you gain weight.

ANDROGEN: Androgens are thought of as male hormones, but women's bodies produce them too, although in smaller quantities. An increase in one androgen, dehydroepiandrosterone, which for simplicity I'll call *androgen,* is one of the first signs of menopause. It is responsible for sending new weight directly to the middle section (helping to create the so-called middle-age spread).

TESTOSTERONE: Testosterone helps create lean muscle mass out of the calories the body takes in. Muscle cells burn more calories than fat cells do, thereby raising metabolism.

During menopause, testosterone drops, causing muscle mass to decrease. This means you have a lower metabolic rate, which means your body burns calories more slowly.

HORMONES AND THE INSULIN, METABOLISM, AND BODY FAT CONNECTION

Various researchers, including those who published a landmark study in the journal *Menopause* in 2010, have found that there is a complex relationship between hormones and weight and one especially vital link connecting insulin, metabolism, and body fat.

Many menopausal women have adhered to a conventional low-fat, high-carbohydrate diet that includes lots of processed foods (pasta, breads, most snacks, etc.). Over time, this type of diet can create insulin resistance. Insulin resistance is a condition in which the pancreas produces insulin but the body does not use it properly. Insulin enhances glucose utilization for energy. Insulin resistance causes the menopausal woman's body to convert every calorie it can into fat—*even* if she's dieting.

When menopausal women are insulin resistant, their muscle and liver cells do not respond properly to insulin. As a result, their bodies need more insulin to utilize glucose for energy. The pancreas tries to keep up with this increased insulin demand by producing more.

Many menopausal women with insulin resistance have high levels of both glucose and insulin circulating in their blood at the same time. The higher their insulin blood levels, the less capacity their bodies have to burn fat.

For women in the perimenopausal stage, weight gain results primarily from widely *fluctuating* estrogen levels. However, for menopausal women, it is the *diminished* levels of estrogen that can cause weight gain.

In all women who are experiencing menopausal symptoms, as their ovaries' estrogen production decreases, their bodies look to secondary sources (including body fat, skin, and other organs) to obtain it. During this period, because their bodies are struggling to maintain their hormonal balance, body fat becomes more valuable as one of these secondary sources.

Because the body is trying to restore the estrogen level while also maintaining bone mass, it needs additional fat cells. The problem is that if a menopausal woman is experiencing stress (not to mention if she's on a low-fat diet plan), her body will go into adrenal fatigue and be in a state of continual struggle to keep body fat, which results in her experiencing little or no weight loss.

When a menopausal woman experiences frequent or regular mental, emotional, or physical stress, her adrenal glands function below the optimal, normal level. For many menopausal women, this adrenal fatigue is most commonly associated with intense or prolonged stress and can change the body's carbohydrate, protein, and fat metabolism. The result? Often, weight gain.

FINALLY, HELP HAS ARRIVED

Another client also came to me after many years of unsuccessful dieting. She had tried the commercial programs, the fad diets on the bestseller lists, the ritzy health clubs, and the celebrity videos.

At 48 years old, 25 years after her first diet plan, she was $15,000 poorer and 70 pounds heavier. By now, the blame was being laid on menopause, and the diet institute's owners, who had profited financially from my client's and many others' fees, were golfing in the Caribbean!

What these patients and many others learned is that there is no diet plan now—nor will there ever be one—that cures overweight. Diet plans do not attack the fundamental problem of the fat person and therefore simply cannot help the menopausal woman.

Menopause Reset! does.

Menopause Reset! Is Simple!

You're about to learn key mind, diet, and exercise techniques that will keep your blood sugar level stable and in the healthy target zone that keeps your body burning fat all day long.

By controlling the physiological effects of perimenopause and menopause with these techniques, you can control menopausal symptoms and their unwanted side effects.

For the menopausal woman, this is revolutionary.

In the past, unless menopausal women were on hormone replacement therapy, there wasn't a lot they could do to positively affect menopausal symptoms.

But *Menopause Reset!* will change all of that.

The key to long-term weight loss success is combining the physiological mechanisms involved in elevating metabolism. *Menopause Reset!* will teach you about the various physiological metabolic mechanisms—what they are, how they work, how they can be controlled and changed, and, most importantly, how to use them to help your menopausal body begin to lose weight.

CHAPTER 3

Step 1: Reset Your Mind-Set!

"Why do *some* people succeed? While others *always* seem to fail?" asked Earl Nightingale, a legend in the personal development world. "Is there a *secret* to success and failure? The answer is yes. You become what you think about."

Nightingale had it exactly right, and that's why *Menopause Reset!* begins with the most important weapon in your fight to get your body back: your mind-set. Your thinking is going to be key to your success.

How you think and what you believe determine how quickly change will happen and how successful you'll be. It's time for you to see your body and life in a whole new way, and to do so, the first step of the program focuses on your mental attitude.

The physiological changes a menopausal woman experiences are tough enough, but when the mental and emotional changes she goes through are added to the mix, coupled with the confusion and stress that go with trying to understand what is happening to her body, a psychological downward spiral is too often the result.

One of the biggest symptoms of this spiral is stress. All of the physical and mental changes happening simply overwhelm most women, and because they've never previously experienced such an event, they have no idea how to deal with it.

As the stress compounds, so do the negative behaviors and actions, which lead to the very thing they simply don't want or need—weight gain.

Many menopausal women don't realize just how big a factor stress is in weight gain during menopause. Stress hormones like cortisol can prevent weight loss because their presence signals to the menopausal woman's body that it should go into an energy-storage mode called the *famine effect.* This occurs when the body thinks it won't receive food again for a prolonged period of long time, so it stores the food it does get as fat (for future energy and survival). This excess fat storage causes weight gain.

Stress can be emotional, physical, and even diet related. While many menopausal women are under tremendous amounts of stress, it's the *prolonged* periods of stress (even as brief as a few weeks) that can lead to chronic inflammation in the body and a metabolic disorder called adrenal fatigue. When this arises, the adrenal glands are too overworked to secrete enough adrenaline, causing body aches, fatigue, sleep disturbances, and changes in the way the body metabolizes foods.

Many menopausal women have found that, try as hard as they might, physiological and nutritional knowledge is not enough to give them the means to successfully change their bodies and symptoms and experiences in the ways or to the degree that they desire.

The good news is, once you know what stress is and where it comes from, you can begin to employ strategies to minimize and eliminate the primary stressors in your life. Making positive body changes will subsequently become much easier.

FOUR STRATEGIES TO START THE MENTAL RESET

My goal is to get your thoughts, beliefs, and actions working in perfect harmony so that unhappy and limiting thoughts and feelings are replaced with empowering new ways to see your body and life.

We'll use four strategies to begin the mental reset.

Mental Reset Strategy #1

HARNESS THE POWER OF DESIRE

*Remember the times and events that made you happiest and
use them to set goals for the future you want.*

The first strategy focuses on core beliefs, goals, and achievement history. I want you to remember the successful times in your life and the feelings that went with them. This is the time when, together, we will introduce and develop a new weight loss core belief system for you based on your past history of successes and achievements.

By focusing on past moments of success and achievement, you can locate "the fire that can lift you higher." In fact, this fire is the beginning of *all* great achievement. It is one of the invisible agents that can turn a person's life from misery to happiness and fulfillment. Its power is tremendous. All of your dreams, goals, and wishes will come to nothing unless you use this awesome power that you *already* possess.

You've got to get fired up about something that you really want to do with your life in order to achieve it! A lot of times we think about something that would really move us deep down inside if we did it. But do you know what happens? We just can't accept the fact that our dreams can and do turn into reality if only we have the desire—and take the actions needed—to see them through.

Desiring something tangible and real, like having the body you've always wanted and being in great shape, and then planning definite ways to achieve that (or any) goal *will* yield results. Desire has the power to transform *it might happen* into *it will happen.*

That power will change your life.

It has been said that 1 person with desire equals the power of 99 people who just have interest. Think about that.

After all, there are a lot of things we're interested in doing, but just how many things do we *desire?* How many things in life do we really get fired up about? There's a big difference between the goals that inspire passion and the aims that are more ho-hum. Recognizing that difference and latching on to the ones that truly light you up will transform your life and your body. You'll be capable of making the move from mediocrity to greatness.

Let's look at a few of the ways you can use the power of desire to turn your fitness dreams (or any other dream or goal you have) into reality.

Think back for a moment to that time in your life when you decided you wanted to change your body. Maybe you wanted to lose weight for a specific event, or simply to be firmer and shapelier. The reason doesn't matter as much as the decision you made and the actions you took.

You went from forming a vision and belief in your mind to turning that visualization and belief into a reality.

From thought, to action, to result.

Beautiful.

And wouldn't it be safe to say, as you look back on the many roads you've taken in your life's journey, that you had no idea of *all* the things you would do; *all* the things you would learn; *all* the energy and sweat you would expend; *all* the hours you would spend dreaming, planning, and working; and *all* the results you would achieve even *before* you began?

You see, inside of you was a vision and a deep desire that something else inside of you told you to follow. You didn't have all the answers—far from it—and you couldn't have told anyone *exactly* what would happen and how, but you believed it would, and that was all that was needed to begin the amazing physical, emotional, and, I daresay, spiritual changes in your body and life.

THINK ABOUT YOUR DREAMS AND GOALS EVERY DAY

See yourself *already* there. Not the way you actually are right now, but see yourself already with the kind of body you've always wanted. Imagine the wonderful feeling of seeing yourself in the mirror and how happy you are. Visualize how good it feels to be in shape and to transform your dreams into reality.

The intensity of your desire will determine how long it will take you to reach your goals.

Just don't give up if the results don't come fast enough. We live in a world where lots of people believe they've got to have everything

5 minutes ago, and if they can't get it now, then they're off to something else.

While others may quit too soon, before they experience success, it is the power of desire that will carry you through the good times and the bad, give you the patience to continue when there used to be impatience, take you over the mountains of success, and help you out of the valleys of disappointment and heartache.

WORDS MATTER

Think of the words that came to mind when I asked you to consider your happiest moments. These words are important. They can serve as your motivators, your points of affirmation.

Words are powerful motivators that can bring inspiration to you and others in a big way.

And the words we say to ourselves either set the limits or destroy any limits on what we will experience and achieve.

Listen up, because you need to hear what I'm about to tell you:

You cannot and will not rise above your words.

Did you get that?
I'll say it again:

You cannot and will not rise above the words you tell yourself each day.

Tell yourself that you're not smart, that you don't get the breaks, that you're too fat or too weak, that you're always broke—anything negative and limiting—and isn't it amazing how life gives you just what you say?

Ah, but begin telling yourself how great and successful you are, how in shape your body is, how the doors of opportunity and good news are always opening for you, and isn't it amazing how life gives you just what you say?

I'm not talking about comparing yourself to others here.

The *only* comparison you should ever make is what you're doing versus what you know you are capable of.

Forget everything else.

The past doesn't equal the future.

Release the Amazing Power Inside of You

Ever think about what you are truly capable of achieving and doing? I'm not talking about what you have done in the past or are doing now. I'm talking about your untapped potential.

Most people are used to doing just enough to keep things going smoothly at their jobs, at school, in relationships, and in anything else that takes effort. After all, the reasoning goes, why do more if you don't need to? And that's the rub.

Little do they know that a little more knowledge, a little more belief, and a little more effort are often the biggest things that separate someone who rises to the top from the rest who settle for crumbs and less than their best.

Here's a wee bit of change-your-life advice: Do just a little bit more than you're doing now, in any area of your life, and the results just might astonish you. The difference between the racehorse that wins the big prize and the second-place finisher that doesn't is sometimes only a split second.

MENTAL RESET STRATEGY #2

THINK OF TODAY AS THE BEGINNING

*Begin fresh, wipe your mental slate clean, and learn to
trust yourself.*

The next strategy focuses on wiping your mental slate clean of the diet and exercise books you've read and the diet and exercise plans you've tried in the past. Our goal is to clear your mental chalkboard of all the misinformation, unworkable beliefs, and previous strategies so it will contain only the things that will work for your menopausal body. This goes for notions you may hold about yourself, too. The past is over. It's time to focus on where you're going rather than where you've been!

Why is it that so much of our daily thinking relates to events, things, and attitudes we have experienced in the past?

If I asked you to estimate on a scale of 1 to 100 what percentage of your mental replay each day is spent on things from the past, what would your answer be?

Most people focus too much energy on the past, which is entirely out of their control, rather than casting their eyes toward the future.

What about workout and diet disappointments that you experienced in the past? How much do you still think about them and, more importantly, how much importance and influence do you allow them to have when it comes to making today's and tomorrow's decisions?

The point I want you to get in all of this is that, while it can be instructive to think about things you've done that didn't turn out like you had hoped or planned, the truth is, they have nothing to do with your body and life *today* or *tomorrow.*

Each day when you wake up, you are given a blank canvas upon which to write anything you choose to do, be, or experience. The more you live your life in the past, the more you're filling up that fresh, new canvas with all the junk from the past, leaving you, at most, only a tiny amount of space for writing the new things you want your life to become.

For most people, that daily new canvas is so filled with yesterday's junk that there's no room to fit anything new and exciting into their lives.

It's time to break the pattern.

FEAR NOTHING

Part of letting go of our past is learning to enjoy today while at the same time accepting lessons from yesterday. In order to base your plans on what you dream of becoming rather than your perceived limitations, you have to confront the emotion that rules many people's lives—fear. It's been said that when we are born, we possess only two inborn fears: the fear of falling and the fear of loud noises. Every other fear you had, have, or will have is learned.

Think about something with me for a moment.

When you were born, you had every possibility of becoming what you wanted to be and doing what you wanted to do. A life of unlimited possibility and greatness was yours.

Then, each year, as you grew older (only in years), you began listening, believing, and accepting—many times without question—the limits your family, friends, co-workers, and society placed on you and the possibilities for your future.

Then it happened.

These limits and these beliefs became your fences. And each year, you accepted more and more of what these people told you, and as you did, those fences began to surround you.

Each year, those fences hemmed you in a little bit more, and you look around now and see that your fences are so tightly constricting your sense of possibility that the best you can do is take a few steps forward and a few steps backward.

Yes, after all these years, because of your fences, you've come to actually believe these limits and imaginary fences are real—even though they never existed except in your beliefs. As a result, your life and experiences are unnecessarily limited.

How amazing is it to think that you were born with an ocean of possibilities—unlimited in abundance and impossible to see its end? And how sad is it that that ocean of possibilities has become a little pool of water?

I've got some news for you: Every single one of those dreams you had as a child and that ocean of unlimited possibilities are still there waiting for you to enjoy—for perhaps the first time in your life. They've *always* been there. You've just chosen not to see and believe them.

When it comes to having the kind of incredible life or body you want, it's never too early or too late to be "what you might have been." Who cares what others think? For so much of your life, you've cared too much about what others think, and look at what that's done to you and how it's made you feel.

The truth is, you were meant to have the kind of life you dream of. Those dreams, those desires, are inside you for a reason.

Step over those imaginary fences and you'll soon find out why.

Be Kinder to Yourself

Some of the toughest battles you'll ever face in life are with yourself. For instance, there might have been a job you wanted that didn't come through, and you beat yourself up emotionally about it. Or maybe it was all the pain and suffering you've faced or are still facing because of all the failed diet and workout plans gone wrong. Maybe you lacked the motivation to stay with the program, or you pushed yourself hard to achieve success so you could show your family and friends that "this time" you were serious, only to have things go wrong—again.

Yet life has a way of neutralizing and healing those pains with time and experience. All of those experiences taught you some very valuable lessons, such as that getting in shape is not about competition, comparison, or proving anything to anyone else. It's about doing it because it makes *you* look and feel good. Because it's good for you, healthy for you, and can help you live longer and experience and enjoy much more of the precious gift of life.

It's about becoming the person *you*—and no one else—want to become and doing things in your *own* way and in your *own* time. Always remember that those in this world who achieve greatness in any calling may be the very same people who have the deepest scars and are therefore capable of feeling even deeper happiness.

TRUST US ON THIS ONE

Part of wiping the slate clean is learning to trust yourself. You are equipped to make good decisions for yourself, and *Menopause Reset!* will help show you the way. But the book you are holding in your hands is just a book. You are the only one who can make it happen. And in order to do that, you have to live by the words of two great philosophers. Johann Wolfgang von Goethe said, "As soon as you trust yourself, you will know how to live." And the venerable sage Ralph Waldo Emerson wrote, "Self-trust is the first secret to success."

Trust: For many of us, it's a word that has paramount importance in how we want others to treat us and how we want to treat them. Sometimes, despite our best intentions, we miss the mark and come up short. But we try, and at the end of the day, that's what matters.

At many times in our lives trust eludes us, especially when it comes to trusting that most important person—ourselves.

Take things as simple as exercise and diet.

For years, we may have listened to the voices of others who proclaimed that they knew what was best for us. And we may even have trusted their advice, only to learn that their words may have worked for them but won't for us.

We sought answers from anyone and anywhere except where our truth resides—within ourselves.

After enough frustration, we took a gamble, made an unsure bet, to actually do something that would change how we looked and felt. Maybe we did it at home or perhaps at a gym or fitness club, but the truth is, we began to trust in ourselves and our ability to make something happen. We took action and the small steps necessary to see where it would lead.

And what a bet it was!

For the first time in our lives, we were seeing and getting results. Real results that weren't just hollow words offered to us by others, but life-changing results.

It was a blast and fun while it lasted. But then, slowly, things began to change.

The results started taking longer and were harder to get to in spite of what sometimes seemed like our herculean efforts.

We began to get unhappy and started looking outside of ourselves, to other things and people, for the answers to our problems.

And this started the cycle of *not* trusting ourselves.

I ask you, could this be where you are right now?

If you answered yes, don't feel bad. You are not alone.

This has been known to occur even in elite athletes, men and women who found the right combination of exercise and nutrition to produce great results for their bodies and then stayed with it and rode that knowledge to every victory they achieved.

But then, once they hit the elite ranks, things got scary for them. They let themselves become unsure of themselves and of many of the things they had done to get themselves to this point in their lives.

They lost trust in themselves.

They replaced that trust with uncertainty and began listening to and following the advice and dictates of those who knew very little about these champions as individuals, but nonetheless were able to convince them (and many others) that they did. The result was often tragedy. And perhaps the biggest disappointment of all is that the athletes didn't listen to what they knew was best for them—they didn't listen to themselves.

They didn't trust the inner voice that said, "Follow me and I'll lead you to every great thing you could ever want or dream of."

And now, so many of them, and countless others in every walk of life you can imagine, live with the regret that "if only I would've, should've, could've . . . "

I'll finish their sentence: "trusted myself more."

Whether it's the exercises you choose, the workouts you do, the foods you eat, or the kind of body you wish to have, you know deep down inside of you that you can trust yourself to make the best choices for you.

Yes, whether it's moving to a new city or country, letting go of an unsatisfying career so you can follow your deepest passion for something brand-new, or tossing from your mental closet all the old frustrations, angers, hurts, disappointments, and beliefs that arose from not trusting yourself in the past, worry no more.

The lighthouse of trust that will guide you unerringly now and for all the days of your future is shining right now and waiting for you.

Waiting for you to follow its beam to the next great chapter in the most important book you'll ever read, the one called *My Life*.

MENTAL RESET STRATEGY #3

[handwritten: Work with a notebook]

KNOW YOUR TRIGGERS IN ORDER TO REDUCE STRESS

Zero in on the things that trip you up to smooth your way forward.

The third strategy focuses on identifying the triggers that sabotage your weight loss success and then giving you powerfully effective strategies to reduce and even eliminate them. Those triggers include:

- **FEELINGS OF DEPRIVATION.** The more you think about keeping yourself away from the foods you love, the less likely it is that you'll be able to do so.

- **BOREDOM.** With more than 10,000 food items in supermarkets, making good choices can feel overwhelming, so you may continue buying the same foods over and over again. It's easy to fall into unhealthy habits and eating ruts. We'll give you the tools you need to develop healthy habits and make good choices.

- **LOW SELF-ESTEEM, POOR MOTIVATION, OR LACK OF SELF-TRUST.** Remember what Goethe said: "As soon as you trust yourself, you will know how to live." *Menopause Reset!* will give you the advice you need to conquer low self-esteem and learn to trust yourself.

- **UNREALISTIC EXPECTATIONS.** Will you lose 15 pounds of fat in 10 days? No, but with *Menopause Reset!* you *will* lose 15 pounds of fat and do so safely and easily, and those 15 pounds will stay off.

Among the strategies we will use to *reduce* or *eliminate* the triggers that may be standing between you and weight loss are to:

- **DEVELOP A LIST OF STRESSORS.** Once we know the stressors (and they are common across a broad spectrum of menopausal women), we can create a de-stressing plan that will provide you with a blueprint for how and when to deal with each stressor throughout your day.

- **JOIN A YOGA OR FLEXIBILITY/STRETCHING CLASS.** Since the mind and body are interconnected, when one is out of sorts, the other tends to follow. You will need to *reconnect* the mental and the physical so that stress-free harmony can be achieved.

- **CREATE A LIST OF THE THINGS YOU ENJOY.** This list may include activities you relish today, or you may have to think back to recall activities or experiences that brought you a sense of fulfillment previously. My goal is to help you remember the things you enjoy and derive meaning from. I want you to bring the fun back into your life.

STRESS: THE CHANGEABLE AND UNCHANGEABLE

When a woman's body is undergoing menopause, it is very sensitive to the influence of stress. By lessening the number and severity of the stressors in your life, you can greatly diminish the impact of (and often eliminate) those stressors that cause weight and fat gain and negative behaviors like bingeing.

In my practice, I've found a very effective way to accomplish this.

We look at the things in your life that can cause you to feel stress (and affect weight gain or loss) and break them down into two kinds: things that are *changeable* and things that are *unchangeable.*

The changeable things are those you have personal control over, like your behavior and your actions. The unchangeable are those you have no control over, such as forces of nature and other people's actions, attitudes, and behaviors. Make a list of each kind.

Let's begin with the changeable.

- Rank these stressors starting with the least important and then escalating to the most difficult ones that you have to deal with.

- Ask yourself how each stressor can be modified so it won't cause stress.

- Create a plan of attack for each one. Write down an action plan that will reduce or eliminate that stressor from your life.

- Set a deadline for when you will have reduced or eliminated that stressor.

- Put your plan into action immediately.

Now let's look at those stressors that are unchangeable.

- Rank the stressors from the least important to the most difficult.

- Create a strategy that will help you change your *perception* of that unchangeable stressor. For example, if someone close to you does things that annoy you and you find yourself focusing on those behaviors the most, a powerful strategy is to *shift* your focus to the person's behaviors you like and enjoy most. Find those things in others that create the best feelings in you and stay focused only on them.

MENTAL RESET STRATEGY #4

SET YOUR SIGHTS AND STAY THE COURSE

Determine why you want to succeed, set goals, and don't let setbacks or slumps get you down.

If your reasons for wanting to achieve what you desire are strong enough, then nothing can stop you from having the success you want. To put it simply: If you have enough reasons *why,* you'll find enough ways to understand *how.*

Before I agree to accept a new patient, I first meet with her at what I call a listening interview. I ask only a few simple questions. My main objective is to listen and understand what brought the person to visit my office.

One of the questions I ask is "What brought you here?"

Many women answer that they want to lose weight and get in better shape.

I then ask, "Why?"

If they answer that they have a wedding to get ready for or the holiday season or some special event that is coming up, I tell them, "I'm sorry, but I won't be able to help you."

You should see their looks of surprise.

"Why?" they usually ask.

"Because," I tell them, "I'm only interested in helping women who want to change their lives beyond just a special event. I want to help women who want to be healthier, feel better, and look great, and not just for the next 2 months—but for the rest of their lives."

And then I say, "So if that sounds like you, then I really need you to think about this and look deep inside for the reasons why you want to eat better, exercise, and do the things that can change your life for the better."

You would be amazed at what such a powerful shift in thinking does for their self-esteem and the results they are now ready to experience.

I want you to experience the same.

Get a piece of paper and a pen and write down the reasons why you are ready to change your body, your eating, and your lifestyle. Then look at the reasons you wrote down. Even if you have just one on that list, but it's a reason you think about time and time again— not simply a desire to change your body because of a reunion, a special event, or another short-term experience—then you have found an anchor for change that will keep you propelled toward that new body and life you so desire.

work in the notebook

Why?

Take Things One Step at a Time

Perhaps one of the toughest things about life is how hard we are on ourselves in trying to make it easier. Not content to take baby steps toward our goals and dreams, we jump in headfirst, giving it everything we've got and hoping to skip many steps that actually are necessary not only for our growth but also for the goal's completion.

You've no doubt heard tales about this tendency. Or maybe you've even experienced it yourself, such as when you started to exercise again. Instead of starting off slow, finding your groove, and allowing your body to adjust, you did too much, overexercised, got too tired and too sore, and quickly lost your motivation to go through that again. It made you miserable, didn't it?

We all have done it, so at least we're in good company. Next time, try this: Do only as much exercise as feels good to your body, and no more. Simply stop, even if you know you can do more. Next time, do a little bit more and stop again.

Keep doing this until you've reached just the right amount of exercise for the right amount of time for your body and goals. You've got the rest of your life to enjoy looking and feeling great. There's no need to try to do it all in one day.

DETERMINE EXACTLY WHAT YOU WANT

Setting goals is key to success. Here are a few things to think about:

- *Determine exactly what you want to look like.* Do you want more muscular arms, a smaller waist, firmer thighs, a flatter belly, and more defined abs? Think about the way you want your body to look.

- *Determine what it will take to get that body.* How many days a week will you work out? What kind of equipment will you use? Free weights, a bike, a stairclimber, an elliptical trainer, a rowing machine? What kind of workout will you do? Be sure that your workout matches the goals you have. What kind of diet should you follow to help you reach your goals? Don't leave anything to chance. Think about everything you'll do that will get you there.

- *Establish a definite date for when you want to have the body you've wanted.* Be realistic. If you're a beginner, then 1 year of training is unlikely to be enough time to turn you into a world-class athlete. So, set short-term goals at first to gauge how your body is responding to the program you have it on. From there, it should be much easier to judge how much time it will take you to reach your big goal.

- *Begin at once to carry out your plans.*

REVISIT, REVISE, AND RESET YOUR GOALS AS YOU GO

Right now is the perfect time for me to remind you—regardless of how fit you may be—that as you become more successful in doing your workouts, in managing your diet, in changing your body's condition and whatever else you do and experience in your life, the tendency will be for you to become satisfied with where you are and to lose the vision and self-trust that got you there in the first place.

Now, I'm not saying that you should never be happy with your achievements. Far from it. I want you to enjoy the fruits of your efforts. You deserve every good and wonderful thing that happens to you. But don't get lazy and complacent and think that life stops where you are.

It doesn't.

The next road is calling you.

So, remember this:

- If you think you've reached peak conditioning, you haven't yet because there's still a little more you can do.

- If you think you've hit your strength limit on any exercise, you haven't yet because there are still a few more pounds you'll be able to lift.

- If you think your body looks its absolute best, you'll be amazed at how expending a little more effort on your weakest muscle area will profoundly affect how you look.

- If you think you've got your diet and nutrient supplementation regimen down to an exact science, you haven't yet because tomorrow you'll be another day older and the ups and downs of life can and probably will change how those old tried-and-true foods and eating habits will work for you.

I want you to get back that vision and unquestionable belief you had years ago when you began. I want you to once again follow it to the next place it wants to lead you.

Trust the vision—always.

You may not know the whys and hows of where it's about to take you, but there is one thing you do know with absolute certainty:

You have firsthand experience of how it changed your life in the past, and you know it can and will do the same from this day forward.

Let it.

MISTAKE YOUR WAY TO SUCCESS

No man ever became great or good except through many and great mistakes.

—*William E. Gladstone*

Accept No Limits

"Where the mind goes, the body follows" is a maxim I've found to be 100 percent true. We can only go as high as our thoughts and our beliefs in ourselves let us. And who sets the limits on those beliefs? We each set our own limits.

Beliefs come from our thoughts, and what we think about, we most certainly bring about. If you have the belief that you'll always be over-weight, out of shape, and look and feel the same, then those thoughts become your limits and you'll never go beyond those boundaries until you change those thoughts to match the changes you want to see happen, the new image of how you want to look and feel.

When my coauthor, Robert, and I first began working out, in our unbridled passion to reach the possible, we made just about every mistake there was to make.

We worked out too hard.

We worked out for too long and too often.

We listened to everyone but ourselves about what the best exercise program for each of us was.

And we valued other people's opinions more than our own and thought they knew how to change *our* bodies and lives better than we did.

Yet, it was through making those mistakes that we began getting frustrated not only by our lack of progress but also by our not following our *instincts* about what we needed to do and when and how we needed to do it, and then just doing it.

Once we realized our mistakes, we quickly changed our actions, listened to ourselves, and followed our own roads. And the results and successes we've realized have been, are, and will continue to be wonderful.

And that's what I want to say to you:

Never fear making mistakes.

Rather, I say, fear *not* making any.

On your journey to build your body and your life into just how you want them to be, you will stumble. You will fall. You will get frustrated.

And you *will* succeed *because* of experiencing those things.

To find the things we want, we first go through the experience of finding the things we don't want.

To find the things that work, we first go through the experience of discovering the things that don't work.

It's an amazingly beautiful process that will bring to us anything and everything we desire as long as we continue to allow life to show us the things we want and what makes us happy by first showing us what things to let go of.

Look at the time you spend exercising and eating nutritiously as priceless time you are spending in your own private laboratory.

Follow your instincts, learn from your trials and errors as you fine-tune your approach, and you'll find just the right things that can bring your life great joy.

CHERISH THE SMALL STEPS

Victory is not won in miles but in inches. Win a little now, hold your ground, and later win a little more.

—Louis L'Amour

As you are moving through *Menopause Reset!* there will be times when you will be very excited about exercising.

There will be times when the next level of strength, tone, shape, and condition you seek will happen so easily.

There will also be times when you won't feel like exercising. You won't feel like going to the gym. You won't have good workouts. You will feel as if you've been wasting time. You will be confused about what's wrong and what you should do. And you will sometimes want to blow off working out to do more fun things.

But you won't.

You won't quit (at least not for any huge length of time) because deep down, you know how good exercising is for you and how it makes you feel when you don't do it.

So, we do what the late, great author Louis L'Amour wrote: We "win a little now," we hold on to the gains and benefits we've been able to experience, and we "hold [our] ground" until the next surge and good result come our way in just a little bit, when we'll be able to "win a little more."

DON'T HOLD TOO TIGHTLY

There's an old saying that always brings a smile and makes us realize the profound truth in it, and it goes something like this:

> *You have to let go of the way things now are to have them the way you want them to be.*

Whether it's your workouts, body, diet, goals, dreams, desires, aspirations, beliefs, wants, or anything and everything else in your life, you first have to let go of what you're now holding on to (since it isn't giving you the results you want), so that the desired thing, the fresh, new, exciting, and *next* thing, can come into your life.

Holding on so tightly to the things that are and have always been leaves no room for the things you now want to find their way to you.

Think about it: You could have all of these wonderful new experiences and enjoyments. They could all be lined up outside your door right now, but they can't come in because your house is packed full of the same old things, in the same old ways, from the same old year after year, that there's simply no room for the new, the different, and the exciting to squeeze in.

Give your body, exercise routine, diet, and life a good shaking up.

It's time to get the "clearing out the mental closet" party started.

Look at all the other parts of your life and do the same. All that most of us need is a push just to get started. Momentum will take over from there.

I'D LIKE YOU TO MEET YOUR NEW FRIEND: "THE AMAZING MR. SLUMP"

Many years ago, a major-league baseball team was in a slump. They started off the year winning nearly every game and then, like a sudden burst of wind, they began losing every game.

The coach tried everything. He gave them good pep talks. It didn't work. He promised them big bonuses if only they'd get back to their old selves and start winning again. Nothing happened.

Finally, on the day of the game that would decide if his team would make the playoffs or not, he did something unexpected.

As the team gathered in the locker room, all dressed for the game, for the first time ever, they waited for the coach.

Never before had the team waited for the coach, because he was the one who was always yelling for them to hurry up and get out to the field. But this time, it was eerie.

The coach was nowhere to be found.

But then the coach suddenly burst through the locker room doors with a wheelbarrow filled with bats.

Every player's bat.

The coach was excited almost beyond words and could barely find them as he tried to explain what had happened.

"The most amazing thing has happened, team," the coach exclaimed as he tried to catch his breath. "The famous spiritual guru Mr. Smith is in the stadium to watch the game today and I took every one of your bats to him and asked him if he would bless them, and he did! He took away any curses and boldly proclaimed that not only will we win today's game, but also that each and every one of you will hit the ball like you never have before!

"It's a miracle, I tell you, a miracle! Now, hurry on over here and grab your bats and let's go. Let's go get 'em!"

The players were stunned.

They looked at each other in amazement and then immediately got all fired up as they rushed over to the wheelbarrow to grab their bats. They had heard the words they needed to hear: The message that had been delivered from on high was that their slump was now *officially* broken.

They rushed onto the field, their newfound power bats in hand, and in less than 3 hours, not only did they win the game by their biggest margin ever, but each player also had more hits and more home runs and had made better plays than at any time any of them could remember.

Was it a miracle?

Or was it belief and a brand-new way of looking at and living their lives?

We all go through slumps.

Not one of us is immune to the ups and downs that life brings us.

We go through slumps in the gym when the good results slow down or stop, or when we don't eat as well as we could.

We go through slumps when it seems like every door we try to open—be it in business or relationships—doesn't want to open no matter how long we try, how much effort and hard work we give it.

But do you know what else is true?

All slumps come to an end.

Some end sooner than others, but make no mistake that if you've been going through just about *any* kind of slump in your life, it's about to end, so you need to get ready for the good news that's about to come your way.

That slump at the gym?

Yeah, it's about to end because you're about to find the new workout and exercises you've needed.

That slump at work?

Get ready, because you're about to receive the good news or inspiration you've been wanting, or maybe it's a new plan and direction that are the next step to a better job, one with better pay and much more opportunity.

That slump in your relationship?

A new day is about to shine on you, because you'll find either the perfect solution to whatever problem or hardship it is that you've been going through or the right decision on taking the next step to bring closure to what's been heavy on your heart for so long.

You see, life has a funny way of testing us whenever we go through slumps.

When times are good, the diet is great and the workouts and gains keep coming and the money and opportunities are plentiful and seem like they'll never end. But it's easy to get full of ourselves and to listen to our egos telling us that we're all this or all that, and we believe the hype.

So, life tries and tries to get our attention when we're going through those good times to tell us that we need to dial it down a notch and get humble again so we can learn our next lessons.

But we don't listen.

We think we know better.

We think we've got everything under control and that we'll come back to that "lesson learning" later.

But we don't.

So life does what it needs to—it gives us a slump.

But life also gives us the directions for getting out of the slump, and here they are:

1. Be honest with yourself and admit that you are in a slump.

2. Humble yourself and get your ego out of the way. Send it on a nice long vacation with instructions never to come back.

3. Remember all the times in your life when you didn't care about power, prestige, title, accomplishments, image, or impressing anyone, when the most important thing in your life was to just enjoy it and have fun. You'll find these were the times when you learned the most, grew the most, and were the happiest deep down.

4. Remember the past successes that *really* meant something to you. From the smallest success to the biggest, see yourself in them and feel again *right now* what it felt like when you were working toward one of those goals and the day you accomplished it.

5. Take those powerful feelings and visions of your past successes and now extend them by giving your mind a brand-new set of dreams and goals—both big and small—that you deeply want to achieve. No limits!

6. Keep from your past only the images of and feelings about your successes. Forget everything else.

7. All that matters right now, at this moment, is where you want to go, what you want to do, what you want to experience, what you want to have and enjoy, and how you will share all of it to help others. See and feel the great feelings you'll have when you reach that dream and share them by helping others.

8. Starting today, think only of who you want to be, and keep thinking about the new you—the one you know you were meant to be.

Forget slumps and don't let them bother you again.

They are simply life's way of getting your attention to tell you that it's time to take a new and better road in your journey on this earth.

Great things are waiting for you.

Amazing things and experiences are just waiting to come into your life for you to have and enjoy.

Make all of your past successes your best friends today. Hold on to them with all your might and never let them go. They are about to guide you to the amazing new life that is waiting for you.

I've got some great news to tell you: All the bats in your wheelbarrow have been blessed.

Go ahead and grab one of them now.

The announcer just called your name.

It's time for you to step up to the plate.

You are about to hit a homerun.

Don't You Dare Quit

Turn on the television and watch any sports star, movie star, or famous singer or musician, and you'll see that they make what they do seem so easy that anyone can do it. But that's because the masters of their art or craft make the difficult seem simple.

Yet, when you read stories about their lives, you'll find that their "overnight" success was 20 years or more in the making, and for many, it's taken an entire lifetime of heartache, frustration, isolation, doubt, discipline, and incredible joy and numbing pain to reach the pinnacle in their fields.

And to think you were bummed out and thinking about quitting when you had a not-so-good workout or the diet went off track. Puts things in perspective, doesn't it?

HOW DOES *MENOPAUSE RESET!* WORK IN REAL LIFE?

Case Study: Mary
Preview the Plan and Move from Mind-Set to Action

Years ago, I had a patient named Mary. Many years had passed since we had last seen each other, but Mary, now 54 years old, wanted to see me. This time, it was for a very different reason: menopause.

As Mary sat in front of me, tears began to well in her eyes as she told me her story.

"It doesn't matter what I do. I simply cannot lose weight. And perhaps if that was my only problem, I could live with it, but not only am I not losing weight, I keep gaining it! Please, Mickey, *I want my body back.* You've got to help me!"

For 2 years, Mary had been gaining weight. She had joined a well-known weight loss program and gotten no results. She had tried to eat well. She had been exercising two to four times a week on her own, doing 45-minute cardiovascular workouts (like walking, using an elliptical trainer, or attending a Spinning class), and two times a week she had a 1-hour session with a private trainer. Yet still she had no weight loss.

On the day I began seeing Mary for the second time, she weighed 160 pounds, had 38.7 percent body fat, and was wearing a size 12.

We began her program by resetting her mind-set.

Mental Reset Strategy #1—Harness the Power of Desire
First, I worked with Mary to help her outline her core beliefs, goals, and achievement history. I wanted her to remember the successful times in her life and the feelings that went with them so we could develop a new weight loss core belief system for her based on her past successes and achievements. This helped her to set goals based on her true wants and needs.

Mental Reset Strategy #2—Think of Today as the Beginning
Next, I asked Mary to completely erase and forget any diet or exercise book, plan, or program she had tried or read about in the past. We needed to clear her mental chalkboard of all the misinformation and

(continued)

Case Study: Mary *(cont.)*

unworkable beliefs and previous experiences so we could write on it only the things that were about to work.

Mental Reset Strategy #3—Know Your Triggers

The third step focused on developing effective strategies Mary could begin to use to reduce stress and the stress-triggered behaviors that were sabotaging her success. Among my strategies for Mary were:

- Developing a stressors list that identified the stressors in her life and creating a de-stressing plan for how and when to deal with each stressor throughout her day.

- Having Mary join a yoga class. Since the mind and body are a harmonious one, Mary needed to reconnect the mental with the physical so that stress-free harmony could be achieved.

- Creating a list of the many activities Mary had previously enjoyed participating in. Our goal was to bring the fun back into Mary's life once again.

Mental Reset Strategy #4—Set Your Sights and Stay the Course

The last step for Mary prior to starting the nutritional and exercise steps was identifying the correct reasons for doing this program in the first place. I asked Mary various questions and looked for the answers that would assure her and me that she was ready to start and succeed and would not fail by default.

- Why you are doing it?
- What are the real, deep reasons for involving yourself in such a program?
- Are the reasons for participating in the program temporary or permanent?
- Are they strong enough and important enough to create the desire for lifestyle changes?
- Are you ready for lifestyle changes and their benefits?

When all of those questions were answered honestly and properly, Mary was ready to start.

I wanted us to focus on three areas of the program that we would incorporate into Mary's lifestyle. We'll learn a little bit more about the hows and whys of diet and exercise in the second and third sections of the book, but just to give you a sense of how we transitioned from resetting Mary's mind-set to resetting her diet and exercise habits, the three areas were:

- Changing how often she ate—I asked her to eat every 2 to 2½ hours

- Decreasing her exercise intensity from the high level she had been doing to a moderate level

- Having her exercise every day instead of two to four times per week

My goals included helping Mary get her body back by regulating her blood sugar level, increasing her body's fat-burning activity, and dialing up her body's daily metabolic rate.

The results were amazing.

By the end of the year, just 7 months later, Mary had reached 146.5 pounds, and she was now at 20 percent body fat and wearing size 8 clothing.

I saw Mary recently, and she is easily maintaining her weight and lower body-fat level, and she can now even get back into her size 6 clothes. She is feeling better, is full of energy, has great self-esteem, and has made a promise to herself—one I know she'll easily be able to keep—that she will never leave this lifestyle of exercise and proper eating habits that I helped her bring back into her life. You can get these same results! Turn the page.

CHAPTER 4

Step 2: Reset Your Diet!

Irving Berlin said, "Life is 10 percent what you make it, and 90 percent how you take it."

Ask yourself: How do you choose to respond to a difficult situation? Do you look at it as a problem, or is it an opportunity? The choice is completely yours. And how you decide can make a huge difference in terms of what you will experience and the kind of life you will create for yourself.

When it comes to changing how you look and feel, just remember that how you eat, what you choose to eat, and when you eat are *your* choices.

You are about to learn how to make the right choices.

FOOD, CALORIES, AND A MENOPAUSAL WOMAN'S BODY

Many menopausal women don't know just how many *fewer* calories their bodies burn as they age due to the ever-decreasing estrogen levels that encourage fat deposits where muscle once was. Nor do they realize how consequential this gradual reduction in calorie burning is for them. As you recall reading on page 16, in the section "The Hormonal Triggers," weight gain during menopause is the most common and distressing symptom for the majority of the female population reaching the menopausal stage of life. And this is due to changes in hormone balance that affect weight control, resulting in a condition we call P-E-A-T.

Progesterone decreases.

Estrogen decreases.

Androgen increases.

Testosterone decreases.

While all four hormones can affect a menopausal woman's body and how it burns and uses calories and its ability to lose fat, estrogen is a key hormone, and here's why: During a woman's fertile phase of life, estrogen is the female sex hormone responsible for causing monthly ovulation. During menopause, estrogen declines rapidly, causing ovulation to stop.

The decreased production of estrogen also plays a major part in weight gain during menopause. As the menopausal woman's ovaries produce less estrogen, her body looks for other estrogen sources. Fat cells can produce estrogen, so her body works harder to turn calories into fat to increase estrogen levels. Unfortunately for her, fat cells don't burn calories the way muscle cells do, and she gains weight.

SAY GOOD-BYE TO THE DIET BEHAVIORS THAT HAVE BEEN HOLDING YOU BACK

Conventional notions about dieting tend to exacerbate these hormonal challenges.

Two of the most common diet behaviors that adversely affect a menopausal woman's body are meal skipping and excessive hunger, both of which can slow metabolism and trigger the body's self-defense mechanism against starvation. When this begins, weight loss becomes difficult, if not impossible.

To better understand why this happens, you need to know what this self-defense mechanism is, what it does, and how to avoid it.

In simple terms, the body's self-defense mechanism against starvation is a physiological instrument that is triggered when you eat *fewer* calories than your body's daily requirement.

When your daily caloric intake falls below 1,000 calories per day for as few as 2 days, it triggers this mechanism. At this point, your body is changing how it functions in response to the decrease in calories. When the self-defense mechanism is triggered, the body automatically reduces its caloric output in order to conserve the few calories you are giving it, thereby creating a major decrease (a slowing down) in the body's daily metabolic rate (DMR). This served us well in our early days as a species; if you don't know where your next meal is coming from, having physiological mechanisms that slow your metabolism and conserve energy is a very good thing. When your next meal is as close as your fridge or the corner store or the supermarket, this mechanism is not so useful.

A similar thing can happen if the body isn't given the fluids it needs at regular intervals throughout the day. If it doesn't receive enough fluid, your body not only holds on to any future fluids it receives (after all, it doesn't know when it will receive any additional fluid), it also holds on to the calories from foods while at the same time *drastically decreasing* your DMR so you slowly burn any calories you need for survival. Being in this metabolic state makes it nearly impossible for fat and weight loss to occur.

Thankfully, none of this will be a problem for you because you are about to reset your diet!

LET THE DIET RESET BEGIN!

If you want to lose weight and fat, then you must reboot your body's fat-burning machine by using the nutrients that are most appropriate for your menopausal body. Food macronutrients such as carbs, protein, and fat, each of which your body processes differently, will affect your caloric output through the digestive process.

In simple terms, here's what you need to know: It takes more calories to break down and digest carbs and protein than fat; therefore, a diet based on a higher intake of carbs and protein than of fat results in a higher metabolic rate.

Menopause Reset! will teach you how to eat these nutrients in the right proportions so your body becomes a fat-burning machine! Unless you've been living under a rock, you are probably aware of the macronutrients we ingest every day. Here's a primer on how they work in your body.

> **CARBOHYDRATES:** The body takes carbohydrates and converts them into something called glycogen. Glycogen is sugar that's stored in the liver and muscles. It is an energy source. The body uses glycogen to contract muscles and to power different organ functions.
>
> **PROTEIN:** The body takes protein and converts it into amino acids, which are needed to repair and replace the cells in muscle tissue, connective tissue, and other tissues.
>
> **FAT:** The body takes fat and, depending upon the composition of the person's diet, either utilizes some of it for energy or converts it into stored body fat.

In order to reset your metabolism, we have to stop the eating behaviors that have prevented your body from burning fat and losing weight.

To give you back your *premenopausal* body, one of the first things we'll do is change how you look and feel by resetting your metabolism back to its premenopausal condition. During premenopause, hormones didn't have such a profound effect on how your body burned food (what's called your basal metabolic rate) or cause your body to store fat more easily, as they do during menopause.

If you were in good shape before menopause, you'll be in even greater shape after your body's metabolism reset is complete.

We're going to use a number of specific principles to begin the diet reset, and one of the most important is the BSR principle.

NOW IT'S TIME TO GET NUTRITIONAL: THE SCIENCE BEHIND *MENOPAUSE RESET!*

To control menopausal weight gain, *Menopause Reset!* targets your body's physiological mechanisms in order to positively affect and elevate your DMR for the day.

Blood sugar (also known as glucose) regulation (BSR) is one of the centerpieces of the *Menopause Reset!* program, and if you wish to *stop and reverse* menopausal weight and fat gain, it is essential that you know how to control your body's BSR. The *Menopause Reset!* plan's principle of BSR will give you tips to follow that will greatly help you to lose the weight you want to and change how you look and feel.

You may be asking, What do weight loss, premenopausal women, and menopausal women have to do with BSR?

A lot!

The scientific findings that link BSR to its effects on menopausal weight gain as opposed to weight loss are well known. Research published in the journal *Menopause* in 2010, for example, shows that a rise in blood sugar results in *excess* insulin in the blood (and therefore in every cell) and *diminishes* the body's ability to effectively use fat for energy, thereby greatly *reducing* your ability to burn fat and lose weight.

Increase in Blood Sugar → Increase in Blood Insulin Level → Decrease in Fat Burning = No Weight Loss or Increased Weight Gain

So what causes blood sugar to rise, triggering an increase in the blood insulin level?

- **MISSED MEALS OR PROLONGED PERIODS BETWEEN MEALS.** Far too many women skip or delay meals. This is a huge mistake for anyone who wants to lose weight. Not eating for 3 or more hours will cause your blood sugar level to drop below normal (to less than 65 milligrams per deciliter), a condition called hypoglycemia. The body tries to remedy this hypoglycemic state by sharply raising the blood sugar the next time food is provided.

This in turn increases insulin production and secretion into the bloodstream.

- **EATING A LARGE QUANTITY OF FOOD AT A MEAL.** The liver breaks down the food we eat into the three major macronutrients: carbohydrates, which are converted into glycogen; protein, which is converted into amino acids; and fats, which are converted into fatty acids and glycerol.

  When excessive quantities of foods are eaten at one sitting, the liver isn't able to break down the food into just glycogen, amino acids, and fatty acids and glycerol. At the same time, the liver increases its production of triglycerides (fat in the blood) and glucose (another name for sugar). When this happens, the blood sugar rises, as does the blood insulin level, which prevents the body from utilizing stored body fat for energy or weight loss.

- **AN INCREASE IN SIMPLE SUGAR INTAKE** (to more than 10 grams per serving). Doing this will raise the blood sugar level sharply, resulting in excess insulin production and secretion into the blood, and will demolish the capacity of the body to burn fat and lose weight.

- **DOUBLE CARBOHYDRATE INTAKE IN ONE SERVING.** The liver breaks down carbohydrates into glycogen. However, when *two or more* starchy carbohydrates (like cereals, breads, potatoes, legumes or beans, pasta, and rice) enter the liver *at or near the same time*, the liver breaks them down into glycogen, triglycerides, and sugar, thereby raising blood sugar and insulin levels and preventing the body from utilizing fats and losing weight. If you eat one type of carbohydrate but have a double serving or some other large portion, your body has the reaction it does to eating a large quantity of food at one time (the second entry in this list), which affects blood sugar and insulin production accordingly.

A DAY IN THE LIFE: HOW BSR AFFECTS MENOPAUSAL WOMEN

Here's a graph that shows how BSR works during a typical day for a menopausal woman.

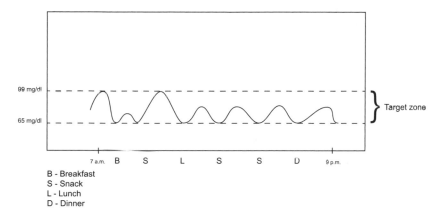

If you look at the left side of the graph (the y-axis), you'll see different levels of blood sugar. Blood sugar is measured in milligrams per deciliter (abbreviated as mg/dl). Normal blood sugar levels for the adult population fall between 65 and 99 mg/dl—the *target zone*, an ideal range for burning fat—but sometimes it will be lower and at other times higher.

Along the bottom of the graph (the x-axis) are the meals and snacks throughout the day. Together, the axes show a typical menopausal woman's blood sugar level throughout a day.

Let's call the woman Janine. Her blood sugar level is shown as a wavy line in the graph. Janine wakes up at about 7:00 a.m., and her blood sugar is normal, between 65 and 99 mg/dl. At that point, she has breakfast. It doesn't matter what she eats right now; what matters is that she eats something, and let's assume she eats a normal breakfast of cornflakes with milk, coffee, and orange juice. Her blood sugar stays somewhere between 65 and 99 mg/dl—that's the target zone on the graph, and ideally, the blood sugar level will fluctuate within that zone all the time.

But then watch what happens.

Beginning 1½ to 2 hours after breakfast, her blood sugar goes up in a wavy line and then back down to the baseline.

An ideal blood sugar curve throughout the day is a wavy line that has only small peaks and valleys, and that's what we are aiming for you to maintain with *Menopause Reset!*

Janine's baseline could be higher, lower, or the same as it was before she ate breakfast depending on what she ate and how much. It typically takes 1½ to 2 hours to digest the food, assimilate it, and eliminate or store it before her blood sugar returns to the baseline.

If she has a snack between breakfast and lunch, she will get another small wave, then a third wave after lunch, followed by a fourth wave after she has a snack.

On this typical day, let's assume that dinner is a little late, so Janine has two snacks before dinner.

The result of the frequent meal feedings throughout the day is a wavy line with *low peaks and valleys.* In essence, that's just what we want: A stable blood sugar graph is what we call *utopia.*

However, *most* menopausal women *don't* eat like this.

Instead, they eat *too much* food.

They ingest *too much* sugar.

They *skip* meals.

They eat the *wrong kinds* of foods in the *wrong amounts.*

They don't eat at the *proper* times.

In other words, the wavy line the majority of menopausal women experience shows what we call the pyramid effect, and it's a condition that can have profoundly negative impacts on their bodies.

For the menopausal woman, the pyramid effect is marked by unregulated blood sugar levels throughout the day. These blood sugar highs and lows affect her body's insulin production in a way that can negatively affect her body's ability to burn fat and lose weight.

Here's why.

Let's assume the typical menopausal woman has breakfast at 7:00 a.m., and after digestion is completed, her blood sugar level returns to baseline by 9:00 a.m., about 2 hours later.

So far, so good.

However, lunch today happens to be at 1:00 p.m., a full 6 hours after her last meal (at 7:00 a.m.).

Remember that it took her body only about 2 hours after her 7:00 a.m. meal to return her blood sugar level to baseline. But because she didn't eat anything for 4 hours after her blood sugar stabilized to normal at 9:00 a.m., by 1:00 p.m., her blood sugar has gone in the *opposite* direction—way down *below* the baseline, putting her body in a hypoglycemic (low blood sugar) state. In a menopausal woman, low blood sugar triggers her body to greatly increase her blood sugar the next time she eats, and this in turn triggers her body to produce more insulin.

That's not what she wanted.

Because of the low blood sugar that put her into a hypoglycemic state, when Janine eats lunch, her body begins manufacturing sugar with the food she takes in, even if she has a nutritious lunch with little or no sugar in it.

Her body's sugar production not only goes into overdrive with that meal, it also continues to operate in this overcompensation mode. Her blood sugar was too low, which caused her body to manufacture more sugar in order to bring her blood sugar level back to baseline. How does this happen? The body manufactures sugar with food and *even within its own body tissues,* just to ensure that it has plenty available to prevent her blood sugar level from dropping to what it perceives to be a dangerous level.

Take a look at the graph below and you can see what happens.

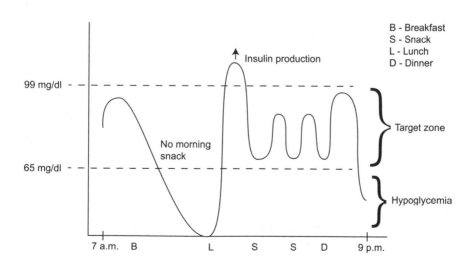

Look at the line after lunchtime. It jumps *way up* over the baseline to about twice the amount it had dropped in the prior 4 hours.

And this is where it gets interesting.

Now, Janine's blood sugar level is way over 99 mg/dl, the trigger point when her body receives the signal that it now has *too much* sugar and needs to do something to correct the situation.

Blood Sugar Regulation Recap

- If blood sugar is not regulated throughout the day, the body cannot burn fat.

- Your blood sugar is at the baseline level when you wake up for the day.

- When you get up and start to use your muscles, your blood sugar level begins to lower. This is why you must eat something within 60 minutes of getting out of bed.

- When you eat, your blood sugar goes up and your body produces insulin to process it.

- Your body goes back to its baseline level within 2 hours.

- The goal is to stop the blood sugar spikes and maintain a shallow wavy line.

- The increase in the blood sugar level above the baseline is proportional to how far you go below the baseline.

- When you feel hungry, you are below baseline.

- You should eat fruits or vegetables *anytime* you're hungry—even if it hasn't been 2 hours since your last meal or snack.

- When your insulin level spikes, your body's ability to burn fat decreases.

- If your body's blood sugar level is constantly spiking, you're putting your body, especially your pancreas, through unnecessary stress.

That's when her body calls on the pancreas.

Why the pancreas?

Because it is the organ that manufactures insulin, and insulin is the primary hormone that helps to regulate blood sugar.

When the menopausal woman's body has high blood sugar, her brain sends an order to the pancreas to go into overdrive and produce a lot of insulin. That insulin, which is transferred into every cell in her body, is on a mission to utilize sugar for energy in an effort to lower her blood sugar level.

Her body will start using the sugar in her bloodstream for energy (rather than burning fat for it) due to the high insulin level in her blood.

And there's more.

About 30 to 45 minutes (no more than an hour) after lunch, her blood sugar level will drop drastically below baseline. While it's higher than it was before lunch, it is still lower than her baseline level.

This yo-yoing (blood sugar going up and down) creates the pyramid effect that results in your having energy and then having no energy, and it helps bring on the feeling of being lethargic throughout the day.

Until now, you simply haven't understood how your eating behavior caused this yo-yoing. With *Menopause Reset!* you will not only understand it, you're going to prevent it.

THE PYRAMID EFFECT
ON MENOPAUSAL WEIGHT AND FAT GAIN

So let's talk about how putting your body into the pyramid effect can affect weight and fat gain.

You need to commit to memory the five behaviors that have a tremendous impact on your physiological mechanisms, the effect they have on your body's blood sugar and insulin levels, and the damage they do to your ability to burn fat.

Controlling these five behaviors will become your key to controlling weight and fat gain and, ultimately, achieving weight loss.

PYRAMID EFFECT #1—SKIPPED MEALS OR DELAYED FOOD INTAKE

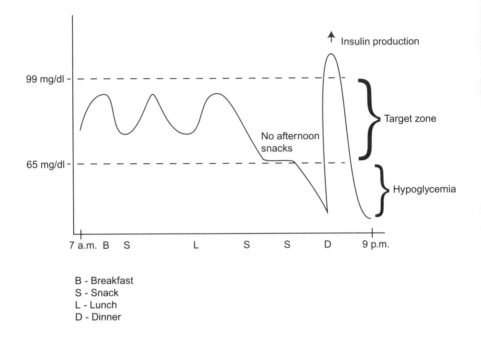

B - Breakfast
S - Snack
L - Lunch
D - Dinner

In this scenario, our menopausal woman, Janine, has breakfast, a morning snack, and lunch, but no afternoon snacks, and dinner is sometime between 6:00 and 7:00 p.m. After having lunch at 1:00 p.m., a full 5 to 6 hours will pass before she eats again.

So what happens?

A repeat of what happened between breakfast and lunch, but in a much more exaggerated way. Janine's blood sugar drops again, but this time, it goes very low.

After dinner, it shoots up twice the amount that it dropped, but then a flood of insulin is secreted by her pancreas, which causes the blood sugar to drop below baseline since she did not eat between lunch and dinner.

To Janine's body, it doesn't matter if it's lunch, dinner, or a snack; anytime she skips or delays food intake, she creates the pyramid effect: Her blood sugar goes up and down throughout the day, and insulin floods into her bloodstream.

Pyramid Effect #2—Increased Intake of Simple Sugars

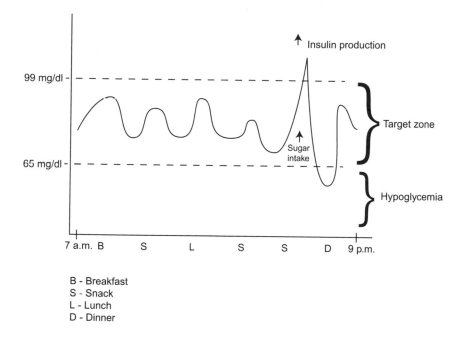

B - Breakfast
S - Snack
L - Lunch
D - Dinner

Let's assume that it is late afternoon and Janine is sitting in her office with a colleague or at home with a friend drinking coffee and eating doughnuts. To her body, coffee and doughnuts are sugars. So what do you think will happen to Janine's blood sugar level 1 to 2 hours after her snack?

Plenty.

Because of the sugar (the simple processed sugar in the dough-nut and the little bit she added to her coffee), her blood sugar will shoot up and her pancreas will secrete insulin again, which will soon be followed by her blood sugar level dropping again—creating another pyramid.

Remember, to your body, simple sugar intake is anything with processed sugar, be it a cookie, ice cream, anything made with juice from concentrate, a hydration drink (these are loaded with sugar), etc. Anything with sugar in it *will* create the pyramid effect.

PYRAMID EFFECT #3—EATING A LARGE QUANTITY OF FOOD

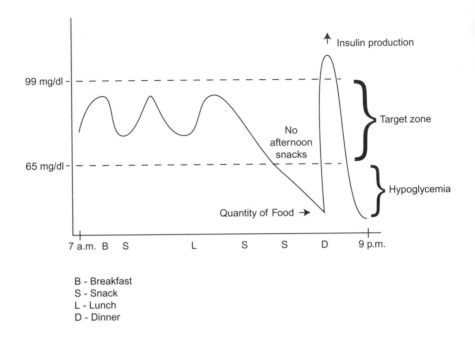

B - Breakfast
S - Snack
L - Lunch
D - Dinner

In this scenario, Janine eats lunch at 1:00 p.m. and has dinner at 6:00 p.m., but no snack all afternoon. But this time she is so hungry, she eats more, which doesn't mean bingeing, necessarily; it may be as seemingly innocuous as going back for a second helping. So what happens to her body after dinner?

When a menopausal woman consumes *too many* calories by eating *too much* food at once, her body converts those excess calories into triglycerides, which are fats in the blood, and glucose, which is sugar in the blood.

Remember this: When you eat too much food, your blood sugar will rise. When your blood sugar is elevated, insulin is secreted to bring it down. Too much insulin inhibits fat burning and weight loss. If you don't control insulin secretion, you are likelier to lose the weight loss battle.

PYRAMID EFFECT #4—INCREASED CARBOHYDRATE OR DOUBLE CARBOHYDRATE INTAKE AT ONE MEAL

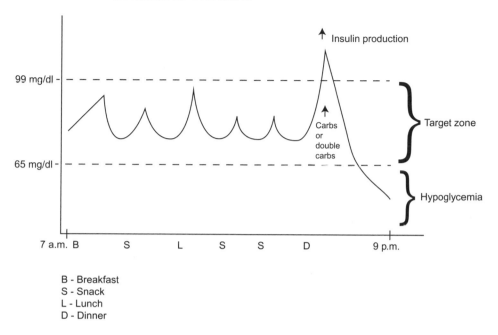

B - Breakfast
S - Snack
L - Lunch
D - Dinner

In this graph, the pyramid effect occurs at dinnertime, but as we've seen, it can happen anytime during the day. This pyramid effect has to do with carbohydrates and how they affect the menopausal woman's body. The typical American diet is loaded with multiple types of carbohydrates in a single meal. And when you go to a restaurant, that's often when trouble begins. The hot, crunchy bread straight from the oven (carb). The salad (carb). The steak and baked potato (carb) or rice (carb), and . . . well, you get the picture.

Carbs, carbs everywhere!

And you eat many of them all at the *same* time.

Big mistake.

Then there are the holidays and special occasions. Barbecues on the Fourth of July, birthday parties, Labor Day picnics, and other gatherings on other holidays and for special events. Hot dog buns, hamburger buns, corn on the cob, pasta salad, potato salad, dessert, and, on top of that, beer.

Double carbs everywhere!

So what happens to your body during events like these? Eating too many carbs at *one* meal has the *same effect* on your body as eating foods in large quantities: Some of the digested food whose components enter the liver gets converted into triglycerides and sugar. The moment you have a lot of or multiple carbs at one meal, you wind up with high blood sugar and then a higher insulin level, and you greatly diminish your body's ability to burn fat and lose weight.

PYRAMID EFFECT #5—LACK OF EXERCISE

The fifth behavior that affects menopausal blood sugar and insulin levels is not nutrition related, but it is an activity.

It's exercise.

For menopausal women, exercise is very important in helping to speed weight and fat loss.

Here's the equation in its simplest terms: Too many calories plus not enough movement equals—bingo!—weight gain.

We want your body to use lots of energy and to pull it from a variety of nutrients within your body, including fats and protein (the least efficient energy sources) and sugar and glycogen (the easiest to access and your body's preferred sources). These are the most important things for you to know: which energy sources from the foods you eat are the most and least efficient, and which sources your body prefers to use.

You'll recall that glucose is the sugar in the blood and glycogen is sugar stored in muscles and the liver. Both are highly efficient energy sources for the menopausal woman's body.

The problem arises when sugar goes unused because your body is not expending enough energy. Your blood sugar gradually rises, putting the pancreas into overdrive to secrete more insulin to keep your blood sugar at a normal level. And as we have discussed, having too much insulin stops fat burning and weight loss right in their tracks. High blood insulin levels diminish the muscle cells' ability to burn fat.

And among menopausal American women, inactivity is an epidemic. Consider this statistic from the US Centers for Disease Control and Prevention's Behavioral Risk Factor Surveillance System survey: During the 6 months before the survey, 85 percent of all menopausal women had not exercised for at least 30 minutes three times per week.

Your goal is to burn energy from morning until night.

With *Menopause Reset!* you're learning how to make that happen.

The Hypoglycemia Pyramid Effect

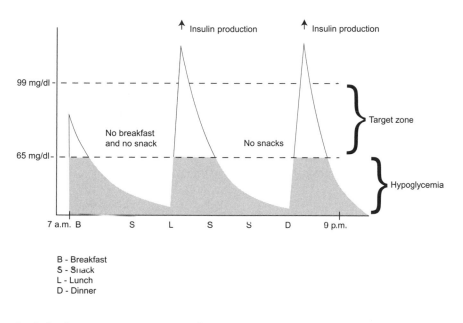

B - Breakfast
S - Snack
L - Lunch
D - Dinner

Let's look at one more pyramid pattern. This one is called the hypoglycemia effect. When your body triggers the hypoglycemia pyramid effect, you have a low blood sugar level. But there's more, as you'll soon read.

As the graph shows, while your body may not remain in the hypoglycemic state all day, it does spend *some* time there, and our goal with *Menopause Reset!* is to keep your body above the hypoglycemic line and stable in the target zone throughout the day.

Symptoms of three kinds occur when your body becomes hypoglycemic. Knowing what these symptoms are can help you avoid hypoglycemia. Take a look at the following categories of symptoms and see if you recognize any of them from your own life.

BEHAVIORAL: Are you tired, fatigued, and lethargic? Do you find yourself procrastinating? Are you moody, or moodier at some times during the day than at others? Are you cranky, irritable, impatient, and bothered by things that never bothered you before? All of these issues could be behavioral changes due to hypoglycemia.

MEDICAL: Do you find yourself experiencing tension headaches, migraines, light-headedness, dizziness, shakiness, or blurry vision? All of these could be responses to hypoglycemia.

NUTRITIONAL: Do you find yourself craving sugar, having an increased appetite, and bingeing? The desire to binge on larger quantities of food (as opposed to eating because you are hungry) could be due to hypoglycemia.

INSULIN AND BODY FAT—STOPPING THE ENEMY IN ITS TRACKS

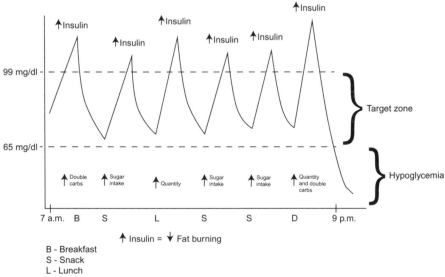

Let's look at one more graph. It shows the correlation between insulin and body fat and how that has a huge effect on a menopausal woman's body.

Look at the bottom of the graph just before 9:00 p.m. It illustrates what we have been saying: There is an inverse correlation between the amount of insulin that is secreted and the body's ability to burn fat. In other words, *the more insulin you have in your body, the less ability your body has to burn fat.*

Simple and powerful.

The bottom line: When you put your body through *any* of the pyramid effects, you will end up with higher insulin levels, which in turn will reduce your ability to burn fat and achieve weight loss.

Fat Cells

- You are born with a genetically determined number of fat cells.

- The smallest fat cells measure 0.01 micron.

- The average person's fat cells are 0.02 to 0.07 micron.

- An obese person's fat cells are up to 0.09 micron.

- When a fat cell reaches 0.07 to 0.09 micron in size, it can split into two fat cells.

- Liposuction can remove 5 million fat cells, but within 3 to 5 years the body reproduces them.

- When you go on a diet plan, your body can lose not only fat and skeletal muscle, but heart muscle too. And when you put the weight back on, chances are that you will put it back on as fat. Then, you'll have more fat, less muscle, and a weaker heart.

- A woman typically gains weight from the bottom up.

- When dieting, a woman typically loses weight from the top of her torso first, then from the bottom.

QUICK REVIEW: MAKE YOUR BODY THRIVE
BY AVOIDING THESE FIVE

So let's recap the discussion. Avoid the pyramid effect by eliminating these five triggers that increase blood sugar and insulin levels.

1. Skipped meals or delayed food intake

2. Increased intake of simple sugars

3. Eating a large quantity of food

4. Increased carbohydrate or double carbohydrate intake at one meal

5. Lack of exercise

RAISE YOUR METABOLISM AND LOSE THE WEIGHT

Women are surprised when I tell them that weight loss isn't difficult. It can be easy, predictable, dependable, and long lasting *if* you follow a few key rules.

Our main goal in the battle to lose weight is to increase metabolism. This is accomplished in two ways: proper nutrition (and proper eating habits) and increased activity.

Some people find it difficult to believe that something as fundamental as metabolism can be changed. But one of the most exciting facts about our physiology is that, yes, we can do various things to change our metabolism. In most cases, we have the ability to raise it (speed it up) or to diminish it (slow it down).

As my 10,000 patients have done, you too can adopt the easy guidelines of the *Menopause Reset!* program, which utilizes the thermogenic effects of food and exercise, correct eating habits, proper food selection, appropriate meal timing, an active lifestyle, and a regular exercise program. All of these factors directly contributed to the very positive changes that occurred in my patients' metabolisms.

THE THREE BIG FACTORS IN AMPING UP YOUR METABOLISM

Three main factors influence metabolism in menopausal women. They are:

1. The thermogenic effect of food (TEF)

2. The body's self-defense mechanism against starvation

3. The differences in the caloric content of each macronutrient and in the way the body processes them

In other words, *you must eat!*

In simple terms, we know that you gain weight when there is more energy intake (caloric intake) than energy output (the calories your body burns), the latter of which is based on the amount of your activity throughout the day.

This is true, but it's not the whole truth.

There are more fundamental questions to be answered.

Are all calories alike?

What affects the rate at which we burn calories?

MAKE IT BURN! IT'S ALL ABOUT THE THERMOGENIC EFFECT OF FOOD

To control menopausal weight gain, along with BSR, *Menopause Reset!* targets one other physiological mechanism: TEF.

Using TEF will help your body stop and prevent weight gain and positively affect and elevate your body's metabolic rate throughout the day to promote fat burning and weight loss.

The TEF physiological effect occurs when the body uses calories to break down the food it receives. And the amount of calories it uses (and how quickly it uses them) is based on the *frequency* of eating, the *quantity* of food, and the *quality* of the food.

Think of it this way: When you eat an apple, you take a bite, and then you have to chew it, swallow it, digest it, break it down into its various nutrients, and finally store it in various places in your body. All of that requires an expenditure of energy. If you skip a meal, you are not encouraging your body to burn energy and calories.

But many women learn too late how to use TEF to their advantage.

A good example is living the college lifestyle. You know how it goes: The schedule from hell, lack of money, parties till dawn, overindulgence in alcohol, and meal skipping all combine to result in the average female student gaining *15 pounds or more* in the course of her 4 college years.

Another example is the premenopausal woman who is gaining weight constantly and believes the only way to lose it is to eat less, skip meals, or not eat between meals. Yet, surprisingly, the end result is weight *gain.*

You must eat and you must eat often—a minimum of six times a day—and doing so will be *one way* to raise your metabolism.

Each time you eat, digesting, assimilating, and using the food your body gets requires energy expenditure. When you eat, many of your body's cells increase their activity. The gastrointestinal tract muscles, which move the food along, speed up their rhythmic contractions, and the cells that manufacture and secrete digestive juices begin their tasks. These cells, and others, need extra energy as they come alive to participate in the digestion, absorption, metabolism, and storage of food.

In other words, *it takes energy to get energy.*

Our bodies burn a certain number of calories simply by converting the protein, carbohydrates, and fats in our food into energy.

Five Ways to Prevent Blood Sugar Spikes

1. Make sure you eat every 2 hours.
2. Keep your intake of foods with high simple sugar content low.
3. Do not eat large portions or second helpings of food.
4. Stay away from having double carbs, or a large quantity of a single carb, in one meal.
5. Exercise every day.

This stimulation of cellular activity is TEF, and it uses approximately *10 percent of the food* you feed your body every day if you eat at least six times a day. If you're eating 1,800 calories a day, you'll burn 180 calories just by eating, without even having to do any exercise.

Eat and burn calories. Don't you love it?!

Understanding this factor will allow you to raise your DMR (daily metabolic rate) *just* by eating correctly.

You need to eat to speed up your metabolism and increase your caloric output. *You need to eat to lose.*

By eating six to eight times per day (to keep your blood sugar and energy levels stable), and eating the proper amount of food and the correct balance of macronutrients within each meal, you'll raise your metabolic rate and caloric output, control the pyramid effect, and increase fat burning throughout the day.

One of the small meals or snacks should be a piece of fruit, and because it is a *natural* sugar, it will actually help to regulate your blood sugar.

Processed, simple sugar, on the other hand, causes sharper increases in blood sugar and can immediately create the pyramid effect.

Natural sugar causes a shallow wavy line (a good thing) in blood sugar, helping you to regulate your blood sugar and avoid the pyramid effect.

My years of work and research with thousands of menopausal women and comparisons of the effects of natural versus processed sugars on their bodies have led me to conclude that as long as the fruit snack has less than 120 calories (80 to 120 calories for each snack is ideal), it will *positively* affect blood sugar because it is a natural sugar rather than a processed sugar. And this has also been found in other research, most notably in a study published in the journal *Menopause* in 2010.

In contrast, when you eat pretzels (which are made with processed, simple sugar) as a snack, you end up with higher blood sugar and triglycerides (which your body makes when you eat too much carbohydrate in the form of starch). The liver converts the carbs into glycogen, glucose, and triglycerides and therefore affects your blood sugar regulation.

What You Need to Know About Your Body's Self-Defense Mechanism against Starvation

What many women don't know is that when they deprive themselves of food, as many commercial diet programs direct them to, the *size* of the body's fat cells shrink, but the *number* of fat cells does not.

As a result, in addition to feeling hungry and deprived, your body thinks you are starving—because you are. It tries to compensate for the reduced intake of food by slowing down how fast you burn whatever food and calories you give it.

This is the body's self-defense mechanism against starvation.

If you reduce your food intake by 20 percent, your metabolic rate can slow down by approximately 10 to 20 percent.

When your metabolism is lower, you burn calories much more slowly, and your body automatically reduces your caloric output.

With the self-defense mechanism against starvation, your body tries to maintain your weight. Even when you go on a calorie-restricted diet, as you start to lose weight, your body tries to compensate on the supply side by increasing your appetite to try to force you to eat more calories and on the demand side by causing your DMR to drop.

This is the dreaded *plateau phenomenon* so familiar to many of us. It really kills motivation as you continue to eat less, but you weigh the same.

If you are on a traditional diet plan that recommends a much-too-low 800 calories a day, the self-preservation system will kick in and prevent your body from burning more than 800 calories per day.

But when you increase your caloric intake again, say to 1,300 calories, your body is going to be stubborn and refuse to burn more than 800 calories.

This is your body's survival mechanism in action.

You see, your body is not convinced that the deprivation time is over, and it's not going to take any chances by throwing calories away.

It's going to *store* those extra 500 calories you're feeding it because it doesn't know when it might receive any additional calories again.

But hope is not lost! With *Menopause Reset!* we can get you out of this cycle.

Two quick and simple ways to do it:

1. Start by eating every 2 hours to move your blood sugar levels back to the wavy line (a good thing!).

2. Eat more than 1,000 calories a day to let your body know that it is no longer in starvation mode.

To illustrate what I've been telling you, let's take the situation of my patient, Janet.

Her eating habits were abysmal. She never took meal timing or food composition into consideration. Worse than that, she was skipping meals.

Janet's self-destructive eating behaviors created a major reduction in her caloric output by slowing her metabolism.

Ah, but watch what happened when we made a few changes.

Janet started eating 1,300 calories a day instead of the 700 calories a day she had been taking in. TEF for the higher-calorie diet was approximately 130 calories a day, versus 70 calories a day for the lower-calorie diet.

That 60-calorie-a-day difference helped Janet burn an extra 21,900 calories in the course of just 1 year.

That sounds like a lot and it *is*, especially when it comes to losing body fat.

Because 1 pound of fat is equal to 3,500 calories, Janet burned about 6.25 pounds of fat using my approach that she wouldn't have if she'd kept to her bad eating habits. Have you ever gone to the grocery store and picked up a 6-pound chicken? Now picture what 6 pounds of fat would look like. It's huge!

And all Janet had to do to experience the wonderful result of losing more than 6 pounds of fat was to *eat more food more often.* Janet is back on the wavy line and her body recognizes it.

Now doesn't that sound great to you?!

I'm hoping you're nodding your head yes, because that's *exactly* what I want you to do.

If you eat six times a day and take in more than 1,000 calories a day, you will bypass, and not have to worry about triggering, your body's starvation self-defense mechanism.

The big lesson here is: Never, ever go on a starvation diet again. And don't you even think about skipping meals.

Doctor's orders!

METABOLISM AND FOOD CONTENT

Okay, so we've talked about the thermogenic effect of food and how to prevent triggering your body's self-defense mechanism. Now it's time to look at the third way to increase your body's metabolism with nutrition, and that is by using the differences in the number of calories each of the macronutrients (carbohydrates, protein, and fat) has and in the way the body processes them.

Your body uses primarily carbohydrates for energy, and it uses those carbohydrates 24 hours a day to keep your entire body running. Your body also needs protein around the clock for tissue repair and growth, cell rebuilding, converting protein into amino acids, and, in very small amounts, for energy.

So what about fat?

You need *some* fat for insulation and lubrication of the internal organs and for blood circulation. However, much of the fat stored in the body is in adipose tissue, a type of tissue that only stores fat.

When do you use this type of fat?

Primarily when you need it for energy, but only during cardiovascular exercise when you get your heart rate up to a certain level and your body has already used up all of the available carbs.

However, most menopausal women are not doing enough of the right kind of exercise at the intensity level that puts them into the target fat-burning zone to burn significant amounts of fat. And that's just one of the problems.

The other comes from eating a diet that's too high in fats.

You probably know the feeling. You have a meal that's high in fat and therefore you might eat less, but you still feel more lethargic than you would have if you'd eaten a meal with less fat.

TURN UP THE CALORIC BURN BY SIMPLY CHANGING THE RATIO OF CARBOHYDRATES, PROTEIN, AND FAT

When you eat different types of food, which you'll remember are composed of macronutrients, your body processes each one differently. Also, your ability to store energy derived from different foods and the caloric/energy cost of storing them are different.

Here's what I'm talking about.

First, in 1 gram of carbohydrate, you consume approximately 4 calories. In 1 gram of protein, you also consume approximately 4 calories. However, in 1 gram of fat, you consume 9 calories.

More than twice as many calories are in that 1 gram of fat.

This should tell you one thing: *If your diet is high in carbohydrates and protein, you can eat double the amount of food for the same number of calories that you would if you ate a diet high in fats.*

If you eat carbohydrates and protein, you can eat more frequently and have much more food but still consume fewer calories than you could if those calories came from fat.

That's huge!

Not only that, but as you now know (and perhaps have experienced all too often), the more fat you eat, the more fatigued and sluggish you feel.

And for good reason.

Fat is not your body's most efficient or first-choice energy source; In fact, as we've seen, the body burns fat for energy only during vigorous exercise. Instead, the body uses carbohydrates for energy first. So if your diet is low in carbohydrates, there's a good chance that you are feeling fatigued and lethargic because your body doesn't have enough to fuel your daily activities, negatively impacting your metabolism and productivity.

But make the switch to a diet with just the right amounts and kinds of carbohydrates and protein and you'll be able to eat more, eat more frequently, be less hungry, and have increased energy.

And there's more.

When you eat a diet rich in carbohydrates, a certain amount of energy is required in order to digest that food, absorb it, and store it.

That means that approximately *23 percent*—plus the 10 percent used by TEF with six or more meals or snacks per day, for a total of 33 percent—of the total caloric intake from carbohydrates is burned in order for the body to store the rest of the carbohydrates for running body functions and generating energy later on.

For every 100 calories of carbohydrates you eat, your body burns 23 of those calories just so it can store those carbs for energy. And you use those calories just by eating—you don't have to do *any* exercise except eating!

That leaves only 77 calories for storage.

Similarly, 23 percent of the calories that you eat as protein must be burned in order to store the rest. As with carbohydrates, your body burns 23 calories just so it can store 77 calories.

This "eating the right foods" thing is pretty great, wouldn't you say?!

But uh-oh. When it comes to fat, it's a completely different story.

While it takes lots of calories from carbs and protein to process and store them, it's not the same with fat.

You only need *3 percent* of the calories from fat to do it.

This means that your body burns only 3 calories out of every 100 fat calories to store 97 calories of fat.

Therefore, your body stores *more* fat calories for every 100 fat calories you feed it, and you feel more fatigued and lethargic and have less energy.

And why would you want that?

Many women say that they find themselves wanting to eat less food when they have a meal that's higher in fat. They think that's a good thing, but it's not.

Even if you eat less food but it's high in fat, your body will store a major portion of those calories.

And since fat is not your body's preferred energy source, where do you think all those extra calories will be going?

Yikes.

Do I have your attention now? Great!

Follow these rules for eating the right foods and you'll always keep your body's fat-burning metabolism fueled and moving at just the right pace.

DR. MICK'S THREE QUICK TIPS TO CREATE THE THERMOGENIC EFFECT OF FOOD

1. Eat a minimum of six times per day: breakfast, morning snack, lunch, afternoon snack, dinner, and evening snack.

2. Reduce your fat intake, increase your carbohydrate intake, and eat sufficient protein. Eat no more than 30 grams of fat per day.

3. Eat more than 1,000 calories every day.

DIETARY GUIDELINES FOR PROPER EATING HABITS

As you're reading this book, I want you to remember that the menu suggestions are not a strict diet. I'm giving you guidelines that you can deviate from, and you can eat anything that is exchangeable.

For example, in the list of breakfast foods that follows, you will see that you can eat half a bagel or a slice of toast or a whole English muffin or a whole pita. You can take an apple or any type of fruit and exchange it for what you like as long as they are comparable in the guidelines.

The food combinations that I've created for you will provide you with two benefits:

First, if you don't deviate from the guidelines, your caloric intake will be somewhere between 1,100 and 1,800 calories per day, which will be a reduction from your current caloric intake. If you are also active (which I want you to be), you will lose weight even more quickly.

Second, using any food combination you choose, as long as you follow the rules, you will not surpass 30 grams of fat per day. As a matter of fact, in most cases you will eat less than 20 grams of fat per day.

One constant to keep in mind is that you should always eat within an hour of waking. What follows are examples of different meals and snacks you can have throughout the day. A 2-week suggested menu follows these general dietary guidelines.

DIETARY GUIDELINES FOR BREAKFAST

Each day, you *must* have breakfast. Be sure not to skip it. Having breakfast each day helps your body stay on the wavy line and off the pyramid effect.

BREAKFAST FOOD CHOICES (PICK ONE):

- English muffin
- ½ bagel
- 1 slice toast

- Cereal with fat-free, 1%, or 2% milk

- Oatmeal with fat-free, 1%, or 2% milk

PLUS (PICK ONE):
- 1 piece of fruit

- 4 to 8 ounces of juice (not from concentrate)

A VERY THIN LAYER, JUST ENOUGH TO FLAVOR THE BREADS, OF ONE OF THE FOLLOWING:
- Butter

- Marmalade

- All-fruit jam

- Cheese

- Cream cheese

SAMPLE BREAKFAST:
- Toasted English muffin

- Marmalade

- Orange juice

- Coffee

DIETARY GUIDELINES FOR LUNCH

You *must* have lunch. Do not skip it. Eat lunch 3 to 5 hours after breakfast, preferably before 2:00 p.m.

LUNCH FOOD CHOICES (PICK ONE):
- Tuna sandwich

- Chicken sandwich

- Turkey sandwich

- Salad and Bread Combo #1: Tuna, chicken, or turkey on a fresh green salad with vinegar and oil, lemon juice, or any low-fat or fat-free dressing plus 1 slice of the bread of your choice

- Salad and Bread Combo #2: Chef's salad with vinegar and oil, lemon juice, or any low-fat or fat-free dressing plus 1 slice of the bread of your choice

- Salad and Bread Combo #3: Greek salad with 1 to 2 tablespoons of feta cheese and olive oil plus 1 slice of the bread of your choice

- Salad and Potato Combo: One of the salads listed above plus 1 baked potato with 1 to 2 tablespoons of sour cream, butter, or salsa instead of the bread

- Soup and Salad Combo: Any type of soup except creamy soups with one of the salads listed above plus 1 slice of bread unless the soup contains pasta or potato

- Pasta and Vegetable Combo #1: Pasta primavera with a small amount of dressing or olive oil for taste

- Pasta and Vegetable Combo #2: Pasta, tomato sauce, and your choice of vegetables topped with a small amount of grated Parmesan or Romano cheese

- Rice and Vegetable Combo: Steamed vegetables mixed with rice blended with a touch of cooking or olive oil with chicken or seafood. Chinese food from a restaurant should be ordered with absolutely *no MSG* (monosodium glutamate, a preservative) and *no salt*.

- Sushi and Salad Combo: Green salad or seaweed salad and 1 to 2 sushi rolls

SAMPLE LUNCH:

- 1 to 2 sushi rolls

- 1 cup seaweed salad

- Water, seltzer, or green tea

DIETARY GUIDELINES FOR DINNER

Again, like breakfast and lunch, you *must* have dinner. Do not skip it.

DINNER FOOD CHOICES:
Fill (but not to heaping) a 9- to 10-inch dinner plate with one of the following.

- Potato and Protein Combo: Baked or mashed potato; 4 to 6 ounces of chicken, turkey, fish, seafood, or tofu (no deep-frying); and a green salad or broiled or steamed vegetables

- Rice and Protein Combo: Rice of your choice; 4 to 6 ounces of chicken, turkey, fish, seafood, or tofu; and a green salad or broiled or steamed vegetables

- Pasta, Vegetable, and Protein Combo: Pasta of your choice; steamed vegetables of your choice; and 4 to 6 ounces of chicken, turkey, fish, seafood, lamb, pork, beef, or tofu

    IMPORTANT: Protein sources may be broiled, barbecued, grilled, or baked—but never fried.

SAMPLE DINNER:
- Broiled fish
- Brown rice
- Asparagus
- Water or seltzer

DIETARY GUIDELINES FOR SNACKS

MORNING SNACK (PICK ONE):
- 1 piece of fruit (the preferred natural sugar) or any vegetable
- 1 banana (an excellent choice, with only 1 gram of fat)
- 1 cup of grapes (less than 1 gram of fat)

THE SNACK IS IMPORTANT—DO NOT SKIP IT!

I will never forget a story one of my clients, the CEO of a major company on Wall Street, told me. Her story proved just how important the morning snack was to her career. Here's what she said happened.

She was attending a very formal morning meeting to sign a big contract with a Japanese firm. Ice cubes are warm in comparison to the atmosphere in that conference room. By 10:30 a.m. there were no signs that the meeting would come to an end anytime soon. My client's digestive system signaled its need for a midmorning snack with loud noises that were heard by all who were in the meeting room.

My dedicated CEO pulled an apple from her bag and, without thinking twice, took a loud, breaking crunch that triggered a change in the meeting. The astonished Japanese delegation and her American co-workers began chuckling as soon as they heard the first bite.

As they laughed hysterically, business moved quickly forward and within the next hour, the multimillion-dollar deal was done. "As long as I live," she said, "I will eat an apple for a midmorning snack!"

I want you to eat every 2 hours to regulate your blood sugar and maximize fat burning.

AFTERNOON/EVENING SNACK (PICK ONE, AND NO MORE THAN 120 CALORIES PER SERVING):

- Fruit or vegetable

- Melba toast

- Crackers

- Whole wheat pretzels

- Rice cakes

- Popcorn without butter or margarine

- Low-fat or fat-free yogurt

- Nuts (almonds are great, but any kind is fine)

Enjoy your snack time, and do not skip it!

MENOPAUSE RESET! 2-WEEK SAMPLE MENU

Here is a **2-Week Sample Menu** featuring 2-hour intervals between meals and snacks. Note that each snack portion should be between 80 and 120 calories.

WEEK 1

Monday

8:00 Breakfast	Yogurt with muesli and mixed fruits (such as berries and mango)
10:00 Snack	Apple
12:00 Lunch	Curry chicken salad on brioche br ead
2:00 Snack	Red bell pepper
4:00 Snack	Nuts
6:00 Dinner	Pasta with pork sausage, broccoli rabe, garlic, and olive oil
8:00 Snack	Berries

Tuesday

8:00 Breakfast	Whole wheat bread with mashed avocado
10:00 Snack	Clementine
12:00 Lunch	Sushi roll and green or seaweed salad with ginger dressing
2:00 Snack	Sugar snap peas
4:00 Snack	Nuts
6:00 Dinner	Broiled scallops, brown rice, and brussels sprouts
8:00 Snack	Orange

Wednesday

8:00 Breakfast	Toasted bagel with scallion cream cheese and lox
10:00 Snack	Mango
12:00 Lunch	Oriental chicken salad with mandarin oranges and toasted almonds
2:00 Snack	Baby carrots

4:00 Snack	Nuts
6:00 Dinner	Pork chop, roasted potatoes, and green beans
8:00 Snack	Grapes

Thursday

8:00 Breakfast	Scrambled eggs and toasted English muffin with goat cheese
10:00 Snack	Banana
12:00 Lunch	Green salad and pasta e fagioli soup
2:00 Snack	Berries
4:00 Snack	Low-fat yogurt
6:00 Dinner	Roast chicken, yams, and green salad
8:00 Snack	Nuts

Friday

8:00 Breakfast	Granola with milk and fresh melon on the side
10:00 Snack	Apple
12:00 Lunch	Low-fat ham and cheese panini and veggies with low-fat dip
2:00 Snack	Red bell pepper
4:00 Snack	Nuts
6:00 Dinner	Chicken, pork, beef, or tofu stir-fry with veggies and rice
8:00 Snack	Low-fat yogurt with berries

Saturday

8:00 Breakfast	Oatmeal with walnuts and raisins
10:00 Snack	Orange
12:00 Lunch	Grilled shrimp Caesar salad
2:00 Snack	Baby carrots
4:00 Snack	Nuts
6:00 Dinner	Pasta with vegetables and chicken breast sautéed with garlic and olive oil
8:00 Snack	Berries

Sunday

| 8:00 Breakfast | Whole wheat waffle or pancake with Greek yogurt, honey, and strawberries |

10:00 Snack	Apple
12:00 Lunch	Omelet with roasted red peppers and mushrooms, sliced tomato on the side, and toast
2:00 Snack	Sugar snap peas
4:00 Snack	Nuts
6:00 Dinner	Rice with pine nuts, broiled asparagus, and salmon
8:00 Snack	Low-fat yogurt

WEEK 2

Monday

8:00 Breakfast	Yogurt with muesli and mixed fruit (berries and mango)
10:00 Snack	Apple
12:00 Lunch	Grilled chicken on a green salad
2:00 Snack	Banana
4:00 Snack	Nuts
6:00 Dinner	Pasta with low-fat ground meat, green peas, garlic, and olive oil
8:00 Snack	Baby carrots

Tuesday

8:00 Breakfast	Oatmeal with walnuts and raisins
10:00 Snack	Clementine
12:00 Lunch	Soba noodle soup and green salad with ginger dressing
2:00 Snack	Red bell pepper
4:00 Snack	Nuts
6:00 Dinner	Broiled shrimp, brown rice, and asparagus
8:00 Snack	Orange

Wednesday

| 8:00 Breakfast | Whole wheat toast lightly spread with peanut butter and all-fruit jam |
| 10:00 Snack | Baby carrots |

12:00 Lunch	Green salad with turkey or ham, blue cheese, cranberries, and walnuts
2:00 Snack	Apple
4:00 Snack	Nuts
6:00 Dinner	Leg of lamb, sweet potato, and edamame
8:00 Snack	Grapes

Thursday

8:00 Breakfast	Fried egg on half a toasted bagel and plum or grape tomatoes
10:00 Snack	Red bell pepper
12:00 Lunch	Tomato and rice soup and ham and cheese panini
2:00 Snack	Berries
4:00 Snack	Low-fat yogurt
6:00 Dinner	Roast turkey, brown rice, and green beans
8:00 Snack	Nuts

Friday

8:00 Breakfast	Cereal with milk and fresh berries on the side
10:00 Snack	Sugar snap peas
12:00 Lunch	Pita, hummus, and veggies
2:00 Snack	Clementine
4:00 Snack	Nuts
6:00 Dinner	Pasta with vegetables sautéed with garlic and olive oil
8:00 Snack	Low-fat yogurt with berries

Saturday

8:00 Breakfast	Whole wheat English muffin with cheese and strawberries
10:00 Snack	Orange
12:00 Lunch	Chef's salad
2:00 Snack	Banana
4:00 Snack	Nuts
6:00 Dinner	Chicken, pork, beef, or tofu stir-fry with veggies and rice
8:00 Snack	Baby carrots

Sunday

8:00 Breakfast	Omelet with jarred roasted peppers and mushrooms, sliced tomato on the side, and toast
10:00 Snack	Apple
12:00 Lunch	Chicken and vegetable fajita
2:00 Snack	Sugar snap peas
4:00 Snack	Nuts
6:00 Dinner	Rice with pine nuts, broiled brussels sprouts, and salmon
8:00 Snack	Low-fat yogurt

NOW THAT YOU UNDERSTAND BSR, HERE'S WHAT YOU CAN DO ABOUT IT

Here are some basic tips:

- Never skip eating breakfast, morning snack, lunch, afternoon snack, dinner, and evening snack.

- Always eat something within 1 hour of waking up. It can be just a small piece of fruit for breakfast.

- Your morning snack must include a fruit or vegetable. Your lunch and afternoon and evening snacks can come from grains, but at least one of those p.m. snacks must include a fruit or vegetable.

- Eat every 2 hours.

- Snacks should be 120 calories or under and have less than 10 grams of sugar.

- Yogurt can be an afternoon snack and can include more than 10 grams of sugar if there is fruit in the yogurt.

- Other good snack choices are pretzels, crackers, breadsticks, and popcorn.

MY OTHER RULES FOR GREAT EATING HABITS

TRY TO AVOID:

- Deep-fried foods

- Second helpings

- Forgetting to eat small meals frequently. Fill up the plate (only once!), enjoy it, and finish it.

ONCE YOU KNOW THE BENEFITS, YOU'LL LOVE THIS NEW WAY OF EATING

Once you start eating this way, you will absolutely love what it does for your body and how it makes you look and feel.

You will not feel hungry or deprived. By not skipping meals, you will keep your metabolism raised and receive many physiological benefits, including lots of energy.

When you eat at least 60 to 70 percent of your daily calories *before* 2:00 p.m., you are less hungry later in the day and able to maximize the burning of calories with activity throughout the day. Eating every 2 hours helps regulate your hunger level, stabilizes your blood sugar level (i.e., it keeps you on the wavy line), increases TEF, and keeps your body burning calories throughout the day.

You're going to find that this is much healthier for you than eating very little throughout the day and then eating a very heavy meal at dinnertime, which will make you sluggish throughout the evening.

Also, by following these nutritional guidelines, you will not surpass 1,800 calories per day, yet you will be eating an abundant amount of foods that are rich in good carbohydrates and protein and very low in fat.

And you'll get no more than 30 grams of fat per day.

THE CALORIE CONNECTION

Let's talk a little about calories.

As we discussed earlier, a gram of carbohydrate, protein, and fat (the macronutrients) contains a different number of calories. And depending upon how much and what proportion of those macronutrients you eat, you will change your caloric intake and therefore your weight gain or loss.

One gram of carbohydrate equals approximately 4 calories.

One gram of protein also equals approximately 4 calories.

Q&A: The Doctor Will See You Now

Any woman going through menopause has questions—lots of them! To save you valuable time and money, here's a *Menopause Reset!* special Q&A with Dr. Harpaz.

Since he's been in practice for more than 20 years and has had more than 10,000 menopausal patients, there's a good chance he's been asked the same questions that are on your mind.

If I have a second helping of food, but it is a small helping, is that okay?
Here's what happens when you have second helpings: You take in *excess calories* your body doesn't need. Try to avoid second helpings if you can.

Is having grains for the morning snack better than having no snack at all?
Yes.

I've heard you say that it is very important to eat within 1 hour of waking up. My question is, If I'm awake but trying to go back to sleep or resting in the morning, should I eat within 1 hour of waking up or 1 hour of getting out of bed?
Eat within 1 hour of getting out of bed.

Should I be concerned about my total daily caloric intake?
The good news is, not if you're following the lifestyle guidelines in this book and eating wisely. People often ask how many calories they need. The answer for each person is different. Unless you have the desire to

---

and can *accurately* track your daily caloric intake, it is very difficult to determine the *exact* number you need every single day. To lose weight, it all comes down to eating slightly fewer calories than your body burns on a daily basis. Once you have reached the desired weight, keep your caloric intake steady (without any further reductions). My advice to you is that you are not a human encyclopedia of calorie calculations, so relax, enjoy, and live well.

Can I eat less than 10 grams of sugar every hour after noontime in addition to my snack? For example, could I have some type of grain snack that has less than 10 grams of sugar at around 2:00 p.m., another snack with less than 10 grams of sugar around 3:00 p.m., a grain or some other snack with less than 10 grams of sugar around 4:00 p.m., and another small snack with less than 10 grams of sugar around 5:00 p.m.?

While small, frequent feedings are great, I advise you *not* to eat numerous snacks, even if they have less than 10 grams of sugar, timed so close together and so consecutively.

How much sugar is in red wine, light beer, etc.?

It all depends on the amount consumed. Check Corinne T. Netzer's *The Complete Book of Food Counts* for the details.

Does less than 10 grams of sugar every 2 hours also apply to alcohol?

Yes.

Is 10 grams of fat per day too low?

Yes. Twenty to 30 grams of fat per day is a good guideline that will meet your body's minimum requirements if you're trying to maintain your weight.

I love homemade applesauce, so if there is no sugar added, can I eat it in place of my fruit snack and can I eat it anytime?

I've got good news for you: Yes.

Are pasta and dumplings considered double carbs?

Yes.

Okay. Are bread and dumplings considered double carbs?

Yes.

(continued)

Q&A: The Doctor Will See You Now *(cont.)*

If a soup has a small amount of pasta and a small amount of corn, do these have significant carb impact or can I eat my bread or potato along with that soup?
My advice is to skip the bread or potato.

Are corn tortilla chips and salsa with real corn in it considered one carb?
Yes.

Which is better, having one large meal or two small meals?
The two small meals and have them approximately 2 hours apart.

What is the average amount of weight lost by your patients?
There is no *average* weight loss. There is a *range* of weight loss, and that's determined by a number of important factors:

1. A woman's genetics and hormonal balance
2. What stage of menopause she is in
3. How she has adapted the *Menopause Reset!* program into her life

How long have they kept the weight off?
The answer is from a short period of time to a lifetime. That is, if they follow the *Menopause Reset!* program as directed and adopt it as their lifestyle, they will never gain the weight back.

How heavy was the heaviest patient you have helped?
One person weighed 325 pounds.

Is there a particular weight loss success story that you're proud of?
I'm proud of every one of my patients. One of the more memorable success stories is a wonderful woman named Arlene who followed the *Menopause Reset!* program, lost more than 90 pounds, and has kept it off for more than 10 years.

However, 1 gram of fat equals approximately 9 calories—more than *double* the amount of calories in carbohydrates and protein.

Simple logic says that if you have less fat and more carbohydrates throughout the day, you will end up with fewer total calories, many fewer fat calories, much less chance of fat storage occurring, and a much higher energy level.

All good things.

So let me give you an example of what I'm talking about.

Beth and Laurie are 50-year-old twin sisters who weigh the same, are the same height, work at the same job, and walk 3 miles a day each.

Beth's caloric intake is 1,500 calories per day, while Laurie's caloric intake is 2,000 calories per day.

So who do you think will gain weight—Beth or Laurie?

It's easy to assume that it would be Laurie, since she is eating 500 more calories per day than Beth. But to answer this question correctly, you need to know more.

You need to know how many of the calories each of the two ladies is eating per day come from fat.

Now look more carefully at their diets.

Beth has a caloric intake of 1,500 calories per day, which is made up of 40 percent fat, or 600 fat calories. Laurie's caloric intake is 2,000 calories per day with only 20 percent fat, or 400 fat calories.

The difference between the two is 200 fat calories per day.

If they continue to eat the same proportions of fat at the same rate for 17 days, Beth will have eaten 3,400 more *fat* calories than Laurie, even though she is eating 500 calories *less* per day. And 3,500 fat calories equals 1 pound of fat.

This means that every 17 to 18 days, Beth will put on 1 pound of fat, unlike Laurie. For every 3,500 calories you consume from fat, if you're not burning any calories of fat by doing cardiovascular exercise in the high-heart-rate fat-burning zone, you will deposit 1 pound of fat on your body. And as we discussed earlier in this chapter, your body burns calories from carbohydrates and protein before it burns fat calories, so fat (whether it's just been eaten or is stored) is the last thing to go.

The conclusion is: For many people, the problem is not so much how many *total* calories they are eating as it is how many calories from *fat* they are eating.

ANIMAL OR VEGETABLE, FATS ARE FATTENING

Fats can be divided into two major categories: animal fats and vegetable fats. Animal fats are in meats, poultry, fish, seafood, dairy products, and eggs. Vegetable fats are in oils, nuts, avocados, olives, seeds,
margarine, etc. Whether it's animal fat or vegetable fat, 1 gram of fat
equals 9 calories.

For the purposes of weight reduction and weight maintenance,
the most important thing to know is that you have to cut down on
all fats in order to reduce the total number of calories that come
from fat.

THE IMPORTANCE OF KEEPING YOUR DAILY FAT INTAKE LOW

The fat content in the average American's diet is approximately
40 percent, which far exceeds what we really need. The body needs
approximately 10 grams of fat in order to synthesize essential fatty
acids. And yet many Americans eat a diet that contains 40 percent
fat. So let's think about cutting this number in half.

And let's try to do it moderately, in a way that will work for you.

Simply adjusting the fat intake in your diet from 40 percent (or
more!) to approximately 20 percent of your total caloric intake would
enable you to actually *slightly* increase the total number of calories
you eat each day with *no adverse effects* on your body.

In a diet that ranges between 1,200 to 1,800 calories a day, the
total fat intake should be between 240 and 300 calories. The average
of the two is 270 calories a day.

If you divide 270 by 9 calories per gram, you find out that someone with an active lifestyle can efficiently use 30 grams of fat a day
and still lose or control her weight. Therefore, *30 grams of fat per
day—or less—is your magic number.*

A GOOD GUIDELINE FOR DAILY FAT INTAKE

For an adult woman weighing 168 pounds who is trying to lose
weight, 10 grams, or ⅓ ounce, of fat per day works wonderfully.

The recommended range of fat intake for weight control is 20 to 30 grams of fat, or ⅔ to 1 ounce of fat per day.

If you can eat fewer fat grams than that a day, that's excellent, but up to 30 grams of fat per day will be okay.

By the way, to help you easily keep track of where you are, just remember that 30 grams equals 1.1 ounces. So, all we are talking about is 1.1 ounces of fat per day.

And remember: Know how many grams of fat are in each portion of food you eat. Then monitor your intake so you do not exceed 30 grams per day, and you will be on the right track to losing weight.

So simple, so powerful, and it works like a charm!

FOLLOW THE TWICE-A-WEEK RULE TO KEEP YOUR BODY ON TRACK

I want to give you a great rule that my patients have found helps them keep their weekly fat and sugar intake right on track.

The following are foods that I recommend you consume no more than *twice per week* for an obvious reason: They have too much fat or too much processed sugar per serving.

Here they are:

- Fried foods

- Poultry: dark meat (white meat can be consumed daily)

- Beef (including ground meat, veal, hot dogs, etc.) and lamb

- Pork (including bacon, ham, sausage, etc.)

- Pizza: Eat no more than 2 slices per week

- Desserts: A serving is 1 slice of cake or pie, 1 small dish of ice cream, 2 to 4 cookies; have these no more than twice per week on nonconsecutive days

- Eggs: Consume no more than 2 to 4 whole eggs per week (though you can have egg whites daily)

(continued on page 97)

Dr. Mick's Holiday Survival Guide:
Follow These Tips to Keep Your Body On Track

With work, holidays, and vacations, it can be easy to get off track temporarily. So, to get your body back to a fat-burning and weight loss machine once again, I'm giving you my holiday survival guide that will keep your diet and body on the road to great results during those special occasions.

Who doesn't like the holidays?! They are a chance not only to see family and good friends but also to eat, eat, eat. And if you've dreaded the almost predictable weight gain that comes from the holidays, it's time to stop worrying.

During the holidays, one of the biggest problems in trying to regulate your weight is maintaining healthy eating habits. Major feasts are a traditional part of celebrating Thanksgiving, Easter, Christmas, the Fourth of July, Rosh Hashanah, Passover, weddings, anniversaries, birthdays, and more. And if we went to only a couple of them a year, there would be no problem. However, many of us attend at least 20 to 30 of these events per year. Add to it that we also dine in restaurants with friends on occasions that are not major events at all, but merely excuses for indulging in good food and pleasant conversation, and the extra calories can accumulate.

So how can you take control of these events and keep your body within the target weight range you desire?

Here's a great example of how to incorporate the principles of *Menopause Reset!* into a major holiday food event like Thanksgiving dinner.

Before the actual meal begins—typically in the late afternoon or early evening, let's say at 3:00 p.m.—maintain your regular schedule, starting with a normal breakfast between 6:00 a.m. and 9:00 a.m.

Eat a piece of fruit for a snack in the midmorning and, believe it or not, at 12:30 p.m. or 1:00 p.m., sit down and eat lunch. Eat a bowlful of rice with vegetables, or perhaps just a bowlful of salad with soup, or any one of your regular lunches.

At this point you will have eaten three times. Your satiety center has received news that there is sugar in your body, and it will slowly suppress your hunger throughout the morning and all the way until 2:00 p.m. When you sit down with the family for Thanksgiving dinner at 3:00 p.m., you literally will not be hungry.

Although you are not hungry, the first thing to do is dish yourself up a bowlful of green salad and a slice of bread. Because you had your breakfast, morning snack, lunch, and now the salad and bread, you definitely are not hungry. Wait 15 to 20 minutes before eating again.

While everyone else is already working on their dinners and, of course, nagging you about not eating, explain that you will eat soon, that you are just taking a break. When the waiting period (15 to 20 minutes) is over, fill up your dinner plate with small amounts of everything on the table, regardless of whether it's a little higher in fat than usual.

There is turkey, sweet potatoes, mashed potatoes, a little gravy, vegetables, etc. Of course, since you're not hungry, you will have a hard time finishing that plate full of food. If you do finish it, that's okay too. But remember one thing from our guidelines: *Never, ever have a second helping.*

Okay, now it's time for the dessert, right?

Not a problem.

An hour or two later, after the table is clean, a delicious array of cakes and pies begins rolling in right in front of you. Yikes! What do you do now?

First, look carefully to see if there is any fruit on the table. If there is, please take a piece of fruit, or whatever there is from the fruit department, and enjoy it. Then take another 15- to 20-minute break. After that waiting period, you can go for your dessert.

Instead of following your usual pattern (i.e., taking a bite of this and a bite of that, a sliver of one cake and then a sliver of another cake), try something very simple. Look at all of the desserts—make sure you see all of them—and select the *one* that you love the most.

It doesn't matter how much fat is in it.

It doesn't matter how much sugar is in it.

Just pick out that special one.

Cut yourself a normal-size slice, like any other guest at the table would. Please eat it and enjoy it without any feelings of guilt.

So what do you think happened to your body—using this new way of eating—at this event?

I'll tell you.

You might have eaten a little bit more than usual, but you really did not indulge. You had breakfast, a piece of fruit, a small lunch, salad, and

(continued)

Dr. Mick's Holiday Survival Guide *(cont.)*

bread. Later on (after the waiting period), you had the dinner plate and you ate a little more fruit, then after another waiting period you enjoyed dessert with a cup of coffee or tea or whatever.

The end result was that you ate just a little too much today—not a lot—and probably more than 30 grams of fat. But its effect on your body will be absolutely minimal. And you won't feel deprived, because you enjoyed (with a slight time delay) all of the foods you loved.

By following the steps described above, you will be able to celebrate with everyone else while maintaining your weight and regulating it in a better way, and sometimes even losing weight.

Exercise on the Day of the Celebration

I also recommend that you exercise on the day of an event, which means exercising in the morning. If you exercise three to five times per week, make sure you count the event day as one of those exercise days.

You might decide to try a different approach and eat like everyone else around the table, but know that this is the only day when you can ignore your new way of eating and abandon your daily fat intake guidelines.

And if you absolutely must have second helpings on these special occasions, then remember this formula to help you keep the weight gain to a minimum: Eat double and exercise triple.

So, let's review your holiday eating game plan:

1. Exercise in the morning, before or after breakfast.
2. Eat breakfast.
3. Eat a morning snack.
4. Eat a regular lunch.
5. At the special dinner, begin with a green salad and piece of bread.
6. Take a break for 15 to 20 minutes.
7. Fill up your dinner plate *once* with small amounts of whatever you like.
8. Choose fresh fruit for dessert, if possible.
9. Take a break for 15 to 20 minutes.
10. Enjoy *one* piece of whatever dessert you like.

Fish and seafood can be eaten every day. Note that for all meats, fish, and seafood, a serving is 4 to 6 ounces. A 157-pound person gets 6 ounces whereas a woman weighing 30 pounds less, 127 pounds, needs 20 percent less, or about 4.8 ounces.

With *Menopause Reset!* you now have the diet tips, tools, and strategies to keep your body looking and feeling fantastic year after year after year.

DIET RESET FINAL REVIEW

You will change how you look and feel by eating in a different way. Begin doing so like this:

- Eat a minimum of six (and up to eight) times per day. These feedings will consist of snacks and main meals.

- Make lists of your favorite protein and carbohydrate foods. You should have at least five different protein foods and 10 different carbohydrate foods to choose from (that includes vegetables and fruits).

- For each meal, mix any one protein and any one carbohydrate food from your lists.

- Each meal or snack will be eaten approximately 2 to 2½ hours after the last one.

- Eat only one carbohydrate per meal. Never have two different carbohydrate foods (or a double portion of one) at the same time.

- Keep your sugar intake under 10 grams per serving.

- Keep your fat intake to no more than 10 grams per meal and 20 to 30 grams for the entire day.

- Each meal should ideally consist of 60 percent carbohydrates (from grains, vegetables, and fruits), 30 percent protein, and 10 percent fat.

- Eat only one serving of each food and one plateful for the entire meal. Never have a second serving.

- Never skip meals or snacks between meals.

THE GET-SMART-QUICK GUIDE TO FOOD LABELS

If you buy food that is high in fat, high in cholesterol, or high in simple sugar, you are already losing the battle. Don't sabotage your success.

In the back of this book, you'll find a bonus section that will teach you everything you need to know about reading a food label. Once you understand what all the numbers and words mean, you will be able to make smart choices and bring home only those foods that can help you lose or maintain your weight. This is half the battle!

Here, for ease of reference, are some highlights. It's the nutshell version of what you need to know about reading labels.

So let me ask you, how much do you know about food labels? If you're like most people, probably not that much. Sure, we've heard about looking on the label to see how many calories a food has, but for many of us, that's about as far as it goes.

It's time we change that. By the end of this chapter, you'll be reading food labels quickly and easily.

The labeling regulations help us identify good foods, their ingredients, and their nutritional values. In 1990, a document from the FDA suggested that consumers demand food that provides convenience, quality, variety, and "health food" attributes. By that same year, supermarkets were introducing an average of 12,000 new food products annually, more than double the number in the previous decade.

Among those 12,000 new foods were lots of "healthy foods" with such enticing descriptions as *low calorie, fat-free, no cholesterol, fiber rich, light, organic, fresh,* and *natural.* Today, the words *lite* and *light* are used to imply that the product has fewer calories; reduced fat; lower sodium; improved texture, flavor, or color; and even a lesser amount of breading.

However, it is indeed rare that we are told about the misleading claims and labels so many foods have. Case in point: Foods that claim *no cholesterol.* Many people will buy these products because they think they're doing something good for their bodies, but that same "no cholesterol" food can still contain a substantial amount of total fat and saturated fatty acids.

LET'S G o LABEL AND FOOD SHOPPING

The majority of foods in grocery stores have Nutrition Facts labels, so I'm going to tell you what to look for and look out for as soon as you begin reading the food label.

The first thing to do is to look for the breakdown given on the Nutrition Facts label. Do not fall for the deceptive headings, titles, or claims on the product's other labels. Then follow these rules:

RULE #1: Make sure that the serving size is one of the standard acceptable measurements: 1 ounce, 1 cup, 1 tablespoon, 1 slice, and 1 each. Make sure you note how many calories are in each serving.

RULE #2: If the product has more than 650 milligrams of sodium per serving, *do not buy it.* Remember, sodium retains water and will slow down and negatively affect your weight loss. In addition, for about one-third of the population in this country, sodium increases blood pressure, and high blood pressure can be a major risk factor for stroke.

RULE #3: This is the fat rule. Find out how many grams of fat are in each serving. Your allowance of 30 grams of fat per day will make it easy to decide just how much you *really* want that food item.

RULE #4: This is the sugar rule. Keep it under 10 grams per serving.

RULE #5: If there is no nutritional information or breakdown of nutritional information on a processed, packaged food, then *do not buy it.* This is a warning sign that the product is high in salt, fat, sugar, or all of the above.

RULE #6: Use common sense. If you follow these rules and use your common sense, you'll be making smart food choices.

One of the fun tasks I give to my patients is to have them go home and pull from the pantry, refrigerator, freezer, and cupboards all of the food products they have.

They then check all those foods out to see if they meet the criteria in the rules I just gave you. If any of those foods are too high in fat or sodium and unopened, they are to take them back to the store. If they are opened or the expiration date is near, then they should throw them out.

MAKING HEALTHY FOOD CHOICES IN ONLY SECONDS

It is time for you to learn the shortcuts that will let you choose a healthy product at the supermarket in only seconds.

Ready? Here we go.

THE FIRST THING TO LOOK FOR: THE NUTRITION FACTS LABEL

Check the product for a list of nutritional information. If it doesn't have any, just put it back on the shelf.

THE SECOND THING TO LOOK FOR: THE AMOUNT OF SODIUM

If the product lists nutritional information, take a closer look. Check the amount of sodium, given in milligrams per serving. If it's more than 650 milligrams per serving, quickly put it back on the shelf and don't buy it.

THE THIRD THING TO LOOK FOR: THE AMOUNT OF FAT

After checking to see that the product contains less than 650 milligrams of sodium per serving, check the number of grams of fat in the product. If it's less than 10 grams per serving, you can buy it.

THE FOURTH THING TO LOOK FOR: THE SUGAR CONTENT

If sugars are way over 10 to 12 grams per serving, do not buy it. Most diet products, especially fat-free products, are loaded with sugar. Too much sugar has a tremendously negative impact on the body's ability to get rid of fat. Just look at how many people swear by fat-free products and yet are still fat or obese. And why is it, if so many people are eating fat-free yogurt, they still have problems getting rid of excess weight and body fat? Be smart: A fat-free or low-fat product *with a high sugar content* is a marketing trap, not a weight loss tool.

THE FIFTH THING TO LOOK FOR: SERVING SIZE

Note the serving size. For example, take a small, 6-ounce tuna can. The serving size is 2 ounces. The Nutrition Facts label refers to a serving size that is one-third of the contents of the can. Also, at that 2-ounce serving size, the 250 milligrams of sodium is below the maximum 650-milligram rule.

So far, so good.

But that is for one-third of the can!

And if you eat the contents of the entire can (very easy to do), then the sodium count zooms to 750 milligrams.

Too high!

If you have a water retention problem or hypertension, make sure that the sodium count is low in every product you purchase.

THE GET-SMART-QUICK GUIDE TO FOOD LABELS REVIEW

1. More than 650 milligrams of sodium per serving? If so, don't buy it or eat less of it.

2. Are sugars more than 10 grams per serving? If so, don't buy it or eat less of it.

3. Are there more than 10 grams of fat per serving? Ask yourself if it's worth buying it when you consider that your total daily fat allowance is 30 grams. My advice: Either don't buy it or eat less of it.

The Reading Labels Review

✔ Look at the serving size

✔ Focus on three key areas:

- Grams of fat

- Grams of sugars

- Amount of sodium

✔ Follow the 10/10/650 rule (per serving):

- 10 grams or less of fat

- 10 grams or less of sugars

- 650 milligrams or less of sodium

✔ When looking at carbohydrate information:

- The total carbs should equal the sugars plus the dietary fiber. If these don't equal the total carbs, use these tips to try to find out why.

  - Look at the ingredients list to see if sugar alcohol or other sweeteners are listed. These sugars often are not accounted for on the Nutrition Facts label.

  - If one of the main ingredients is rolled oats or other grains, the unaccounted-for carbs are probably from grains and are therefore okay.

  - Foods like meatballs may contain bread, and if so, you should carefully consider whether to have them since the bread may result in double carbs.

- Any word in the ingredients list that ends in -*ose* is a simple sugar (i.e., fruct*ose,* dextr*ose,* etc.).

- 1 ounce of sugar = 28 grams

- 1 tablespoon of sugar = 11 grams

CHAPTER 5

Step 3: Reset Your Movement!

One extra degree makes all the difference.

When you boil water, it is only hot up to 211°F. But at 212°F, just 1° more, water boils, and when water boils it creates steam, and if you rustle up sufficient steam, it has the power to move a locomotive pulling 100 cars.

Think about it: Just 1° extra has all that power!

And, it's that 1° of extra effort that separates the great from the greatest in business and in life.

Consider this:

> When you total the number of winning strokes for all the major golf tournaments over the last 25 years, the average margin of victory was less than three strokes.

> Over a 10-year period, 1.54 seconds was the average margin of victory in the Indianapolis 500 car race. And those 1.54 seconds earned the driver in second place an average of $657,000 less than the first-place finisher.

When it comes to your life and the things you want to experience, it's time for you to turn up the heat.

To get what we've never had, we must do what we have never done, and so many times, that means making just 1° more effort.

So let's talk about Step 3—Reset Your Movement!—and how you can add just 1° of extra effort to get amazing results by targeting your metabolism with movement and exercise.

IF YOU'RE LOOKING FOR A PERMANENT WAY TO KEEP THE EXCESS WEIGHT OFF, THIS IS IT

The simplest way to speed up your metabolism is by increasing your regular daily activity and exercising a little more each day. A fantastic benefit of exercise—besides making you look and feel great—is that it will increase your metabolism for up to 12 hours postworkout! Exercise will also increase your muscle mass while decreasing your body fat, and that can positively change your ratio of lean body mass to fat, which will increase your metabolic rate throughout the day.

Evidence proving that exercise is the most effective way to control weight permanently is rapidly accumulating. Exercising and leading an active lifestyle do wonders for the body's metabolism.

The truth is, our bodies simply were not designed for the sedentary life or for eating sparingly to make up for a lack of activity. Our instinct is to consume enough energy to support a good deal of physical activity. Nature didn't envision desk jobs, televisions, computers, or automobiles when putting the human body together.

Exercise is one of the most important factors in increasing metabolism. It is an incredibly important factor in gaining the benefits discussed throughout this book. Exercise is also the main thing that helps you regulate your weight loss or maintain your weight once you have achieved your ideal weight, and that's why I want all of my patients to make regular exercise a part of their lives for the rest of their lives.

And you too!

I've told you that Americans are eating fewer calories now than in 1900, yet more of us are overweight than ever before. One of the biggest reasons for that is that we're doing less activity.

Technology just keeps making our lives easier. We have greatly reduced the energy-consuming demands of work. Labor-saving devices are as common in the home as in the factory. Fewer people do manual labor. More people are in white-collar jobs, sitting at desks in front of computers all day long.

For too many people, physical exertion on the job is unnecessary. And it is amazing to discover the lengths people will go to in order to avoid the slightest bit of activity in spite of its obvious health benefits.

In addition to proper eating habits, for *all* of my patients, having an active lifestyle has been the answer to changing their bodies and lives.

It is also the answer for getting a low body fat level, good muscle tone, a higher metabolism, stress relief, and many other benefits. Not engaging in such a lifestyle deprives you and your body of so many benefits and rewards.

And yes, I know how hard it can be sometimes to *start* exercising and becoming active. My patients tell me all the time.

But they do it, and once they do, they *never* look back.

For us to get your body to the place where it will once again burn fat and food optimally, we're going to get you moving in some very specific ways.

Our goal is to use the thermogenic effect of exercise (TEE) to keep your body's fat-burning and energy-using metabolism elevated throughout the day, and we're going to do it by using the *Menopause Reset!* program's physiological movement dynamics.

They are:

- The *mode* of your activity, meaning what kind of exercise you do

- The *duration* of your exercise, or how long you spend exercising

- The *frequency* of your exercise, or how often you exercise

- The *time* of day you exercise (a.m. versus p.m.)

- The *quantity* of your exercise, or the amount of exercise you do each day

- The *type* of training you do (strength training using free weights, body weight, or exercise machines, or cardio exercise)

- The *sequence* of your exercises, or what exercises you do first and which other ones follow

- The *intensity* of your movement, or how easy or difficult you make the exercise

KNOW THY MISTAKES AND AVOID THEM

Before we can change your body with exercise, you must know what are the biggest mistakes that can hold you back and the most effective ways you can avoid them.

While millions of menopausal women start exercising each year, millions of them stop because of the lack of enjoyment, motivation, and results. We are about to change all of that by telling you about the biggest factors that sabotage exercise and weight loss and the step-by-step things you can do to prevent them from happening.

Those factors are:

- Not committing to regular exercise

- Not having the right reasons for exercising

- Using the wrong mode of exercise to meet your goals

- Exercising at a too-high intensity throughout your regimen

- Doing an exercise routine that is too short or too long

- Exercising at the wrong location or time of the day

LACK OF EXERCISE

Any activity, movement, or exercise requires muscle contractions. To power these contractions, the body utilizes blood glucose as one of its energy sources. A lack of activity and exercise *decreases* sugar utilization and causes a slow *rise* in blood sugar, which in turn creates an *excess* of insulin in the blood (and therefore in every cell and tissue) and *diminishes* the body's ability to effectively use fat for energy, thereby greatly *reducing* its ability to burn fat and lose weight.

Your metabolic rate—also called your daily metabolic rate (DMR), which is the body's total caloric output throughout a day, including all rest and activity— is determined by two components: your basal metabolic rate (BMR), which is the minimum caloric output needed simply to sustain life, and your exercise metabolic rate, which is your total caloric output (beyond the BMR) that results from activity and exercise. These can vary drastically depending upon your actions and whether you are living an active or inactive lifestyle. As I've seen in the thousands of women I've helped throughout my years of practice, there is no doubt that *leading an active lifestyle is the most powerful factor in increasing metabolism and, therefore, your caloric output throughout the day.*

Rev Your Fat-Burning Metabolism with Movement

Menopause Reset! gives you the specifics on how to rev up your fat-burning metabolism by using the most-effective workouts and prolonging the postworkout metabolic spike.

Guide to Revving Your Fat-Burning Metabolism with Movement

Here's your brief guide to maximizing your metabolism!

EXERCISE IN THE A.M. Research published recently in the journal *Best Practice and Research Clinical Anaesthesiology* found that a morning exercise session positively changed the metabolic rate for the rest of the day. A p.m. session loses some of that benefit. If you exercise in the morning, you will reap the benefits throughout the day.

MAKE YOUR CARDIOVASCULAR EXERCISE SESSIONS LAST AT LEAST 30 TO 45 MINUTES. Research published recently in the *American Journal of Preventive Medicine* found that in the first 12 to 15 minutes of any exercise program, the body utilizes more glucose and glycogen than fats for energy. Only after 15 to 20 minutes of exercise is there a transition—from glucose and glycogen to fats—in the body's primary energy source. This is due to the fact that in the first 15 minutes of any exercise routine, the body uses mostly sugars for energy and very little fat. The bottom line: The menopausal woman who needs to lose weight will burn fat by exercising for longer.

USE THE THERMOGENIC EFFECT OF EXERCISE. This physiological mechanism is a *postexercise* effect. Studies show that there is an increase in the metabolic rate of 5 to 10 percent *after* exercise, and it can last for 8 to 12 hours. TEE *alone* can produce an astonishing 10 to 12 pounds of weight loss in 1 year.

The Exercise Effect: Move More and Be Rewarded with a Faster Metabolism

Once you embrace the idea of being more active, we guarantee that you will love how it makes you feel. And there are many other benefits, too!

EXERCISE LOWERS THE RISK FACTORS FOR:

- Cardiovascular disease

- Diabetes

- Osteoporosis

- Stress-related illnesses

And there are many more. Moreover, you can maximize exercise's benefits with aerobic exercise. We now know that this type of exercise (also called cardiovascular, or cardio, exercise) has the most dramatic effect on the metabolic rate.

It increases our caloric output during the exercise session by increasing our metabolism.

If you do cardiovascular exercise at the right level—in your target heart rate zone—you are also increasing your body's ability to utilize fat for energy to contract your muscles.

The Attitude Effect on Raising Your Metabolism: Get Moving and Get Burning

Women are surprised when I tell them that their attitudes can be a *huge* influence on their bodies' metabolic rate.

How can the right kind of thinking do that?

Easy.

If you see yourself as an active person, you will become more active.

Since your daily metabolic rate (DMR) is mostly based on what you *do* throughout the day, be honest and ask yourself how often you:

- Drive rather than walk

- Take the elevator or escalator rather than the stairs

- Take a parking space that is the closest one to the store

It's all about being more active, and the more active you are throughout the entire day, the better it is for your body (and metabolism) and the better you will feel.

The world we're living in is constantly simplifying our lives so we have more time to do the things we really want to do.

But even though we have so much free time, if we don't include the right amount of activity in our lives, it can keep us lazy and fat.

Think about it.

You're at the point in your life now where you're no longer struggling and you're making good money that allows you to hire people to do the things you used to do yourself, like mowing the lawn, cleaning the house, or whatever.

Yet, it was many of those now-hired-out activities that helped keep your metabolism running quicker and more efficiently.

It is these kinds of activities that can keep your metabolism running higher throughout the day and keep your DMR higher. The body needs energy to perform those activities, and increasing your body's caloric expenditure will help you lose weight and keep it off.

I always tell my patients that having the right attitude toward being more active and then taking action by becoming more active is the first and best way to increase your metabolism.

The more you do, the more you lose.

The numerous positive life- and body-changing benefits of this new way of thinking and doing will be of enormous importance to you.

You may have learned that to find your target heart rate, you subtract your age from 220 and then multiply that number by a percentage. For years, that was the accepted standard (and it still is). But there is a more accurate way to determine your target rate if you really want to get the best results.

I use the Karvonen equation.

Since our goal is for you to exercise at moderate intensity in order to achieve the best fat loss benefits, let's use the Karvonen equation to find your target heart rate.

Let's say, for example, that you are 50 years old. We begin by subtracting your age (50) from 220, which gives us 170.

We then subtract your resting heart rate—let's say it is 70—from 170, and that gives us 100. (To find your resting heart rate, take your pulse before you get out of bed in the morning.)

We then multiply 100 by 50 percent to determine the lower number in your target range and then multiply 100 by 70 percent to find the upper limit of your target range (50 to 70 percent is a good exercise intensity range for fat burning), and that gives us 50 and 70. Now, we add your resting heart rate of 70 back into each calculation, and that gives us your target heart rate range of 120 to 140.

Cardiovascular exercise in this intensity range can help rid your body of fat.

THE POSTEXERCISE EFFECT ON METABOLISM

Looking at exercise only in terms of burning a certain amount of calories in a certain period of time gives you an extremely limited perspective on the importance of exercise in weight loss and weight control.

If the average adult woman walks 2 miles, she will burn approximately 200 calories per mile.

It is also true that these 200 calories are equivalent to the bagel that walker had for breakfast, and therefore it may not seem worthwhile to exercise.

But it is, and here's why.

Excess postexercise oxygen consumption—think of this as another way of measuring the effect of exercise on your DMR—is simply an increase in demand for oxygen that occurs after your exercise session and affects metabolic rate and caloric output. It drastically increases your DMR, which remains elevated for some time after you've finished exercising. If you exercise in your target heart rate range for about 45 minutes five times a week, there will be an increase in your body's metabolic rate that lasts for anywhere from 8 to 12 hours after you've finished.

Did you get that?

For as long as 12 hours after you've exercised, your metabolism is still elevated. Research by Kazunori Ohkawara, PhD, and colleagues that was published in the *American Journal of Clinical Nutrition* in 2008 found that just *30 to 60 minutes of cardio each day* will drastically increase your caloric output and fat burning in comparison to exercising for less than 30 minutes. In addition, the researchers found, vigorously exercising for 30 to 60 minutes will elevate your body's DMR for an average of 10 hours and possibly for as long as 12 hours after you've exercised. If you exercise for an hour five times a week, that amounts to about 50 hours, or 30 percent, of your week with a raised metabolism compared to none if you didn't do any exercise.

So after your workout, your body's engine is still ticking faster, requiring more energy, even if you're sitting on the sofa. Your body continues to burn more calories by needing extra oxygen postexercise than it does normally.

Sounds great, right?

You see, when you exercise, it's not only about how many calories you burn during your session, it's also about what goes on in your body *after* you've finished.

The Importance of Muscle

Exercise has tremendous and multifaceted benefits for your body over the long term. One of those very positive effects is that your BMR—your basal metabolic rate—is increased due to a change in your body's composition: Exercise tends to improve your ratio of muscle to fat.

What so many women don't understand is how important it is to have strong, shapely muscle on their bodies. It not only looks good, it's also very healthy for you. Muscle is metabolically active, and it takes calories to maintain it. That keeps your metabolism running faster than it would if you didn't have that muscle.

When you lose weight by restricting the amount of food you eat, you lose fat tissue, water, *and* muscle.

And when you regain the weight, in the end you wind up with proportionately *more* fat than you lost due to the fact that you have regained fat and water, but *not* the muscle you lost.

And if you are not exercising during the time you are putting on weight, you are not gaining muscle, and therefore, you become proportionately fatter. You will have much more fat in your body than you did when you started. And you will also have *less* muscle, which makes your bone density and your lean body mass (LBM) lower than they were before.

This has a drastic negative effect on your metabolism! Not to mention that you will also be weaker because you have less muscle and less power.

THE LEAN BODY MASS–TO–FAT RATIO AND WHY IT'S SO IMPORTANT TO YOU

When I ask my patients if they know their LBM-to-fat ratio, they look at me like I'm from another planet.

No worries.

I'm about to tell you just what it is and why it's so important to you.

- One cell of muscle weighs much more than one cell of fat.

- One cell of bone weighs much more than one cell of fat.

- LBM includes muscle, bones, and organ tissue.

You increase your LBM by toning your muscles and increasing their weight, which also elevates your bone density.

By reducing body fat, you reduce its weight in the body. The higher your LBM-to-fat ratio, the higher your metabolism, and the more calories your body has to burn in order to move that muscle from one place to another place.

Therefore, *the goal is to have a higher LBM-to-fat ratio to increase your metabolism.*

This physiological fact is borne out by the fact that for the overweight people among us, it is easier to stay fat or to become fatter than it is to lose fat and become leaner. Leaner people have a higher DMR and a higher LBM-to-fat ratio. Fatter people have a lower metabolic rate so it's much more difficult for them to lose weight.

And then there's the conundrum of thin or lean people being able to walk in the mall eating a whopping ice cream cone and still maintain their weight.

It's not fair, I tell you.

But here's the reason why it's true: The more you increase your LBM (your muscle), the higher your metabolism throughout the day. So, the effect of exercise is not limited just to when you exercise for those 30 to 60 minutes; the metabolic spike goes far beyond that.

A REAL-WORLD SCENARIO

Let's take a look at an example illustrating the LBM-to-fat ratio: a woman who weighs 160 pounds and has 40 percent body fat and 60 percent lean body mass.

The 40 percent body fat weighs 64 pounds. The 60 percent LBM weighs 96 pounds. This particular woman's LBM-to-fat ratio, then—determined by dividing 96 by 64—is 1.5.

The same woman, a few years later, has slimmed down to 132 pounds, achieving a 28-pound weight loss. She has also reduced her body fat to 21 percent, which now represents 28 pounds of the 132 pounds. Her LBM is 79 percent, which represents 104 pounds out of her 132 pounds. When we divide 104 by 28, we get an LBM-to-fat ratio of 3.71.

The difference this change has made in her metabolism is incredible.

The change in this woman's LBM-to-fat ratio means she burns *two and a half times more* calories due to her increased metabolic rate.

That means that if you just sit where you are and burn 100 calories, this woman will burn 250 calories in the same amount of time without making any more effort than you are.

A *big* difference!

And it doesn't take an expensive gym membership or fancy exercise machines to make changes in your body's metabolic rate and in the way your body looks and feels.

Consider this: Just 2 miles of walking burns up 200 calories.

If you do that five times a week, in 3 years you will have significantly changed your lean body mass. That will make an amazing difference in your body's resting caloric output, which has a very positive effect on your DMR.

WOMEN AND MEN ARE JUST DIFFERENT

What I just described to you also explains the body composition and metabolism differences between the genders. A man and a woman who weigh the same and eat the same diet may find that the woman gains weight while the man simply maintains his weight.

On the flip side, if they're both on the same type of diet program, the man will lose more weight than the woman will in the same amount of time.

Why?

Women have a lower metabolic rate than men because of the difference in their body composition. Women generally have a much lower lean body mass and a much higher percentage of body fat than men.

That's why I want you to get comfortable with the idea of adding more muscle—the right muscle in the right places—to your body.

Muscle accounts for about 90 percent of the metabolic rate at rest, during exercise, and postexercise. If you lose muscle mass, you lose a powerful calorie-metabolizing tool, and your need for calories will go down.

To make matters worse, if you are not eating properly or frequently enough throughout the day, that dreaded weight gain will too often be the end result.

If you exercise regularly, it will stimulate the synthesis of protein and muscle growth. At the same time, it will help reduce body fat by using it to produce energy for the working muscle. When you exercise, you are not only getting rid of unwanted fat but also increasing the amount of muscle in your body. This improves the ratio of muscle to fat, and that will result in an increased metabolic rate and more energy expenditure.

Yep, that means burning more calories more quickly.

Let me tell you how adding muscle helped my patient Janet.

To change her metabolic rate, I advised Janet to implement a combination of correct eating habits providing the needed nutrients for added muscle and an exercise program for body fat reduction that would help her gain more muscle. By using this program, she changed her LBM-to-fat ratio.

Janet reduced her body fat by 25 percent and increased her lean body mass. This elevated her BMR and DMR, both of which are important factors in helping her maintain her current weight.

Another patient of mine, Roberta, a college dean, had been living a sedentary lifestyle, and as noted by Audrey Bergouignan, PhD, and Stéphane Blanc, PhD, in a review article published in the *Journal de la Société de Biologie* in 2006, she was much like approximately 70 percent of the American population. I knew we would have to raise her metabolism. Making exercise part of her lifestyle was one of the ways I decided we would do it.

Today, Roberta is at her local health club 4 mornings a week, and she says her newfound energy level—the result of exercise and a good diet—is giving her more energy than she ever imagined she could have.

The good news is that Roberta's metabolism is now at a level that allows her to consume normal amounts of food six times a day and maintain her 28-pound weight loss with ease.

IT'S TIME TO GET HONEST WITH YOURSELF

Now that you know just how important increasing your daily activity level is to your metabolism, body, and life, I want you to answer some questions. In order to evaluate your activity level and exercise habits, pick a normal (or average) week in your life to record all of your activities. You will be evaluating how active you really are—in other words, are you moving your body throughout the day or not? Be honest with yourself.

- How active are you in general?

- Do you have an active job or a desk job?

- Do you drive to most of the places you go to?

- How active are you at home?

- Do you come home at night and collapse with the newspaper in front of the TV, eat dinner, watch a few shows, and go to bed?

- Or do you help clean the house, play with the kids, and take care of the garden?

- Do you exercise at all?

- If so, how much, for how long, and how many times a week?

- What kind of exercise do you perform: aerobic or cardiovascular; weight training or a strength program; tennis; skiing; soccer?

There are so many simple ways to increase your daily activity: walk more, drive your car less, take the stairs more often instead of using the elevator, etc.

Let me give you a few great ways to exercise that are simple and produce very beneficial effects on your metabolism.

The first thing you must do prior to starting any exercise program is to check out your medical condition with your physician. Remember, it is your responsibility to make sure that exercise is safe for you. Check with your physician or physiologist to see if you need medication to control any untreated conditions and to determine if it is safe for you to begin an exercise routine.

To reduce the risk factors for heart disease, to achieve weight and fat loss, and to improve your cardiovascular conditioning, I recommend doing some kind of aerobic exercise. An aerobic exercise program will increase your caloric output and your fat burning.

So, for higher fat loss, as well as for the reduction of risk factors, cardiovascular exercise is the recommended type. That means that the activity mode should be an aerobic activity like walking, jogging, or cycling.

PUT ON THOSE SHOES AND START WALKING

I love walking, and it is the first exercise I recommend to my patients. We were born to walk.

So, get yourself a good pair of proper walking shoes, put them on, and start walking. Walking is the least expensive and the easiest way to begin a cardiovascular exercising program.

Of course, if you can afford to invest in cardiovascular exercise equipment for home and that's the kind of exercise you enjoy, then go for it. But you don't need to. Walking is the ideal start.

So what about joining a health club so you can use their cardio machines?

Statistics show that most health club newcomers quit within 2 to 3 months. That means they are using their gym memberships for only 8 to 12 weeks. Ever wonder how a 30,000-square-foot facility with limited exercise machines can have more than 2,000 members? Can you imagine what would happen if even half of them showed up at any given time? The health clubs know most people will join and then soon quit.

Keep in mind that joining a health club can be a great idea for some, but not for all. Similarly, most of the home exercise machines can produce results for many of us. However, my experience with many of my clients has taught me that over time, these machines become just another piece of dusty furniture or a major laundry-hanging rack. For drying my towels, I prefer a clothesline to a $1,500 exercise machine.

Your best bet is walking.

So, first, get your doctor's approval to start exercising. Then, before you begin walking, or any exercise program, you need to make the decision that there will be no excuses.

You must make the decision to consider exercise a normal part of your lifestyle—as habitual as brushing your teeth in the morning. Remember, even four visits to the mailbox at the end of the driveway is better than sending the dog to pick up the mail, and it can be a real key to your success.

EXERCISE FREQUENCY

The recommended frequency of exercise is daily, as in seven times a week. You eat every day and you have a metabolism to take care of, so help your body by giving it daily exercise.

Of course, the more you do—within reason, of course—the better your results will be. I'd rather have you begin your program by exercising daily for 10 to 15 minutes and building up to 30 to 45 minutes instead of doing 1- or 2-hour marathon sessions that'll quickly burn you out and increase the chance for injury.

No need to rush things.

For my patients, I've found that *daily exercise produces results that are faster than and superior to those seen with exercising only three or four times a week.*

THE BENEFITS OF REGULAR EXERCISE REST BREAKS

Every once in a while, give yourself a break and skip a day of exercise in order to reduce your risk of developing long-term injuries such as tendonitis; problems with your Achilles tendons, knees, or hips; and lower-back pain. Taking a regular rest break will give your body time to recuperate and prepare itself for the next workout.

I suggest that you *take off at least 3 consecutive days every 4 weeks.* The break is just long enough to get you rested, but not long enough to lose the benefits and conditioning of your regular exercise. This performs two primary functions.

1. Even when you're making great progress, it makes you even more motivated. You see and feel your body making terrific progress and you want to keep going, but you stop and give your body those few days of rest. On the 3rd day of rest, you will be so looking forward to and excited about getting back to your exercise plan that your motivation level will be sky-high. That's the kind of strategy that will keep you exercising consistently and feeling great for life.

2. Forced rest days (i.e., 3 days off in every 4 weeks of exercise) will help your body keep from becoming burned out and injured by overuse. Many women exercise too often for too long and do not take enough days off so their bodies can heal, recuperate, rebuild, and strengthen. I think you'll enjoy just how well 3 days off in every 4 weeks of exercise will work for you.

How Long Should I Work Out For?

As for how long you should exercise, I suggest 30 to 60 minutes for each session.

If you are just starting your exercise program, your goal is to work up to this amount. So, start with 5-, then 10-, and then 20-minute exercise periods, building endurance slowly. Continue building up until you get to anywhere from 30 to 60 minutes. Eventually, you can work yourself up to 45 to 60 minutes—the recommended duration of a good walking workout.

As you build yourself up, the better and stronger you will become. And the longer you exercise beyond 30 minutes, the more fat you will burn.

At the beginning of any exercise session, your body is more likely to utilize more glycogen (from carbs) than fat as an energy source so your muscles can contract. Therefore, during the first 20 minutes of exercise, you are utilizing lots of glycogen and some fat.

When you keep exercising past the 30-minute point, your body switches to stored fat as a main source of energy. If you exercise for 30 to 45 minutes, and eventually up to 60 minutes, fat utilization increases, and therefore body fat and weight reduction increase, too.

Keep in mind that the duration and frequency of your exercise are the most profound catalysts for your body's fat reduction.

And it's very important that you take those forced rest days (i.e., 3 days off in every 4 weeks of exercise). However, let me give you an example comparing the power of only walking to running a marathon. Walking 3 miles a day, 7 days a week, 50 weeks a year (allowing 2 weeks of vacation) adds up to more than 1,000 miles of walking for the year. This is comparable to doing approximately 40 walking marathons in 1 year, and I have yet to meet anyone who has walked in 40 marathons who is overweight.

EXERCISE INTENSITY

In order to gain the maximum benefits from exercise, you should exercise to the point where you're mildly to moderately sweating and your breathing is mildly labored. Moderate exercise uses 50 to 70 percent of your maximum exercise capacity, and its benefits include improvements in cardiovascular function and increased fat burning, which is what the menopausal woman is after. In comparison, you reach an intense exercise level when you're using 70 to 85 percent of your maximum exercise capacity, and it yields increased cardiovascular benefits. Intense exercise, in many cases, should be prescribed by your family physician or by an exercise physiologist based on your performance in an exercise stress test.

If you do get the okay from your doctor after a stress test and you start walking on your own, the guideline above still applies: exercise to the point where you are mildly to moderately sweating and your breathing is mildly labored.

One way of determining how hard you can really push yourself is to take the "talking test." You want to be sure that you can talk to people who are exercising with you. If you're out of breath and unable to talk while you are exercising, then there's a good chance you are overdoing it, so dial down the exercise intensity until you reach the point where you are able to speak while you exercise.

Once the exercise activity you're doing becomes easy and you don't have to exert much effort, then you can slightly raise the intensity level by walking faster, walking for longer period of time, taking longer strides, taking shorter strides at a quicker pace, holding a pair of light weights in your hands, or attaching weights to your waist, ankles, or wrists.

When starting an exercise program, begin slowly, gradually increasing the frequency, duration, and intensity—not all at once. Allow your body to gradually adjust to the changes and the new demands you place on it, and it will reward you.

It is generally recommended that if you are more than 35 years old and have not exercised for a while, you should consult a physician first. Follow your physician's advice, and always use your common sense. And remember, walking is the easiest, most natural, and least expensive way to exercise.

A final word: If you do not like the word *exercise* and all the things it is associated with (i.e., exertion, sweating, etc.), then just think of it as an activity, like feeding the birds or having sex or doing anything else that creates more of a happy, positive image for you.

You have my permission to call it anything you want, just as long as you do it!

JUST WHAT YOU'VE BEEN WEIGHTING FOR

You should see the reactions on women's faces when I tell them that I'm creating a strength-training workout for them that includes weights.

My goodness, the shock on their faces and the fear that shows in their eyes that they might become too big or too muscular is priceless. Heaven forbid!

But soon, those looks change to smiles after I tell them they *won't* get too big, they *won't* get too muscular, and they *won't* get too strong,

Exercise Recap

- Exercise every day for at least 30 minutes.

- If you like to bicycle, just remember that sitting on the bike for 60 minutes is equivalent to approximately 30 minutes of walking for the same given heart rate.

- Body versus gravity is the key to exercise, and in our opinion, walking is the best activity that uses it.

- When cardio training, remember that when you are exercising in the 70 to 85 percent target heart rate zone, your body uses more sugar than fat. When exercising in the 50 to 70 percent of your maximum exercise capacity, your body burns more fat than sugar.

but they *will* get shapelier and healthier and love even more the skin they're in once they see and feel the results they'll get with a good strength-training program.

And so will you.

Perimenopausal and menopausal women who add strength training to their weekly exercise routine can expect:

- A higher metabolic rate, greater caloric output, and greater fat burning due to the improved LBM-to-fat ratio

- A decrease in their osteoporosis risk due to the gradual, long-term increase of LBM

- An increase in total body strength

- A decreased rate of injuries due to increases in LBM and total body strength

The great thing about strength training is that you can do it anywhere and you don't need to join a gym to experience its amazing health benefits. You pick the place, time, and environment that will work best for your life.

QUICK LIST OF EFFECTIVE AND INEXPENSIVE EXERCISE EQUIPMENT FOR YOUR HOME OR OFFICE

You don't need expensive equipment to get great exercise results. Here's a list of the basics you simply can't go wrong with:

- Dumbbells (2, 3, 5, and 10 pounds, two of each)

- Jump rope

- Swiss (balance) ball

- Exercise mat

Remember that the strength training is in *addition* to your cardiovascular program, not a substitute for it. I want you to include *both* in your weekly exercise program. You will find that the benefits of each separately and when they are combined will be tremendous.

MENOPAUSE RESET! EXERCISE PROGRAM: GUIDELINES TO FOLLOW

The menopausal woman's body responds best to a very specific physical training regimen that is carefully designed around her delicate endocrine system. During menopause, a woman's hormonal balance (i.e., the changes in her body's testosterone, estrogen, and progesterone levels) is hypersensitive to physical stressors and demands placed on her body.

The wrong kind of strength training can produce horrible consequences that include increased body fat, elevated cortisol levels, and significant weight gain. The right kind of training will produce marvelous results. Our goal is to have you exercise at the intensity level that will produce just the right amount of stimulation to make your muscles and cardiovascular system stronger and more toned, but not so much that it overtaxes your muscles, connective tissue, central nervous system, and hormone levels and produces negative effects and results. In other words, we want you to get your body back to just where you want it to be!

Case Study: Allison's Story

When Allison first came to see me, the first thing I noticed was that she didn't need to lose weight. At 51 years of age, Allison was postmenopausal and one of the few lucky ones who do not gain weight as part of the menopause changes.

However, Allison's bone density suffered from the changes in her endocrine system, and her risk for osteoporosis was very high.

My strategy to help her and reverse her risk was threefold:

1. I had Allison eat on time for better regulation of blood glucose and optimal digestion of nutrients.
2. We created an eating plan that ensured that Allison consumed the right ratio and amount of calcium in foods and supplements.
3. I developed a comprehensive exercise program that emphasized strength training to develop stronger and more toned muscles, strengthened tendons, and increased bone density throughout Allison's body.

Six months later, we were amazed at the changes.

Her bone density had increased by 1.9 percent, and just 1 year after starting, Allison's bone density had increased by another 5.9 percent and reversed her risk for osteoporosis.

I see many women—peri- and postmenopausal—who are suffering from a lack of strength and a risk of osteoporosis as well as from the other effects of menopause. It's one of the reasons why I want to get them involved in some type of strength-training program early on. I've seen firsthand how the right kind of strength workouts can dramatically change a menopausal woman's life for the better.

To help you do that, we're going to change your menopausal body by moving it in a different way. And we begin doing so like this:

- During the first 30 days on the program, do only cardio training to help you burn fat and change your body's lean body mass–to–fat ratio. A good thing!

- You will exercise for a *cumulative* minimum of 30 to 60 minutes of cardio each day. In other words, you do not have to do all of your cardio exercise at once. You can split it up by doing some cardio in the morning (before breakfast, on an empty stomach, is an ideal time to spark your metabolism), some in the afternoon, and some in the early evening. The goal is to do a minimum of 30 minutes to a maximum of 60 minutes of cardio activity throughout the day.

- During the first 30 cardio-only days on the program, you will exercise every day, with no days off from training. Our goal is to help you build a body with a strong foundation, and one of the key components to that foundation is to strengthen your cardiovascular system so it will benefit from both aerobic (the cardio exercise you'll be doing) and anaerobic (the resistance exercise you'll soon add) training.

- The optimal time for you to exercise (if your schedule permits) is in the morning, between the hours of 5:00 and 11:00. However, the most important thing is that, regardless of what time you are able to exercise, you *do* exercise. It's all about the thermogenic effect of exercise! Remember: Morning exercise is better than afternoon. Afternoon exercise is better than evening. And evening exercise is better than none.

During each exercise session, get the maximal fat-burning effect by exercising in the target heart rate zone of 50 to 70 percent of maximum capacity. Since our goal is for you to exercise at moderate intensity in order to achieve the best fat loss benefits, let's use the Karvonen equation to find your target heart rate.

Let's say, for example, that you are 45 years old. We begin by taking the number 220 and subtracting your age (45) to get 175.

We then take 175 and subtract your resting heart rate, and let's say it is 65. That gives us 110.

To find the heart rate range you're shooting for, we multiply 100 by 0.5 and then by 0.7 (because 50 to 70 percent is a good exercise intensity range for fat burning) and those two calculations give you the numbers 55 and 77. Now we add your resting heart rate of 70 back in, and that gives us your target heart rate range of 120 to 142.

So, cardiovascular exercise in this exercise intensity range can help rid your body of fat.

- After 30 days of cardio-only exercise, your body is now ready for you to add strength training. On day 31, you will begin strength training three times per week (i.e., Monday, Wednesday, and Friday, or any 3-day-per-week combination that allows 2 days of rest between workouts and 3 days of complete rest, meaning no strength or aerobic exercise, after your third workout for the week). You will use a combination of free weights, machines, and body-weight-only exercises.

- You will strength-train by doing multiple sets (three or more, depending upon body part) of high-repetition exercises (in the 12- to 25-rep range, depending upon body part) using light weights of no more than approximately 30 percent of your maximum 1-rep ability. **Important note:** We recommend going to your favorite gym or health club to have a fitness professional help you determine your maximum 1-rep ability.

- Beginning on day 45, you will use a double-split training routine on at least one workout per week. Ideally, this workout will include 30 minutes of cardio training with your workout being completed by 11:00 a.m. and 30 minutes of strength training with your workout completed by no later than 3:30 p.m. Using this powerful technique no more than once a week, research shows, will give you even greater results than you would get without using it because of its ability to doubly stimulate your body's endocrine system and metabolism.

- In all strength-training workouts, your pace should be quick, with only 20 to 45 seconds of rest between sets and less than

Are You Salt Sensitive?

The blood pressure of one-third of the US population is sensitive to the effects of salt. To test whether yours is, do the following:

1. Relax for 3 to 5 minutes and then use a blood pressure monitor to check your blood pressure (BP).
2. Put ¼ teaspoon of salt on your tongue and allow it to dissolve for 1 minute.
3. Recheck your BP.

If the reading goes up by 10 to 15 points, you are salt sensitive; if it goes up or down by about 5 points, you are not salt sensitive. If you are salt sensitive, watch your sodium intake carefully.

Exercise = sweat = salt loss. The more you exercise, the more salt your body will need.

90 seconds of rest between body parts. We have found that this exercise pace produces consistently great results for the menopausal women who follow it.

MICKEY AND ROBERT'S SMART EXERCISE AND DIET TIPS FOR EXTRA SUCCESS

When people start hitting the iron, they do so for a lot of reasons. Perhaps it's to get bigger and stronger. Maybe it's to lose weight. It could be to rehab after an injury and get themselves back in shape. All well and good, mind you. However, what far too many people neglect—and oftentimes, they don't realize it until years down the road—are the terrific benefits of making smart aerobic training (i.e., cardiovascular exercise) a must-include component of your total fitness program.

It's easy to see the superficial aspects of your effort—the muscles pumping, limbs moving, and all that good stuff—when you're working out, but "under the hood" is where the things that really matter and can give you longer life and optimal health take place.

When you're hitting it big-time aerobically, here's what's happening on the inside:

- You breathe more deeply and faster to get more oxygen into your bloodstream.

- Your heart beats more quickly to ensure that the increased oxygen intake is distributed throughout your body.

- Your small blood vessels dilate to deliver the extra oxygen to your tissues. (Over time, as you become more aerobically fit, you even develop more of these vessels.) This also helps your body to rid itself of such things as lactic acid and carbon dioxide.

- Your body experiences a huge feel-good endorphin release.

OTHER BENEFITS

- Tired of catching colds and the flu and getting sick? Add aerobic workouts to your week and watch your immune system strengthen.

- Want to lower your chances for getting high blood pressure? Aerobic training can help you do that.

- Want to cut your chances for getting colon or breast cancer? Adding aerobic training will help you do it.

- You say you don't want to develop heart disease or have a stroke? Then start doing more aerobic training.

- Worried about your cholesterol and triglyceride levels? Add aerobics to your workouts and watch your HDL level (the one you want to be higher) go up and the bad LDL (the one you want to be lower) go down.

Ah, but I can hear you now. "Yeah, I know I should probably do

---

Remember the Last Experience

Always remember the mental principle of the Last Deposit. It states that you remember most strongly the last experience you had doing anything you do. That's why when it comes to your workouts and exercise, you should always make sure to end your exercise session with something positive, like that extra rep, extra effort, or anything else that leaves you feeling good about yourself. It'll be the first thing you'll remember when it comes time for your next exercise session.

---

more aerobic training, but I don't have time and it's hard to get motivated to do it."

Here are even more reasons why aerobic training is important:

- It strengthens your heart.

- It helps keep body fat levels low and your body looking (and feeling) better.

- Aerobics can help to keep your blood sugar stable so you don't experience those huge spikes of lots of energy and then the deep pits of no energy (of course, proper nutrition is the foremost way to control this, but aerobic exercise is right behind it as support).

- And yes, aerobic workouts give you much more stamina for those fun activities you like so much outside the gym (you know what I'm talking about, so let's keep it clean here, folks).

ADVICE FROM THE OLD SCHOOL

Over the years, one of the questions I am often asked is how people can avoid overtraining. It's time for me take you to the "old school" for some answers.

For women, workout success has two big potential enemies: undertraining and overtraining. It helps to know the warning signs of each.

Let's start with undertraining.

To keep it really simple, you're undertraining when you're either not doing enough training or not training at the intensity level needed to produce noticeable changes in strength, size, or other aspects of your appearance or any discernible internal changes, like lower blood pressure, reduced stress and hypertension, improved mood, better digestion, etc.

For many women, getting on the right kind of workout plan for their goals and level of ability and increasing the intensity of their effort often is all that's needed to break the undertraining cycle.

When it comes to overtraining—that is, when you're working out too intensely, too often, and not giving your body time off for sufficient rest and recuperation—things get a bit trickier.

Seeing and feeling great results are things that most people don't want to give up. You reach goals as the result of a lot of hard work, time, sweat, and energy. However, unless you time your training cycles correctly, those gains can stop quickly.

Some of the common overtraining signs are:

- Irritability

- Lack of sleep

- Poor digestion

- Nervousness

- Strength plateau or decrease

- Longer recovery times after workouts

- Injury

And the last one, injury, is the one that, more times than not, is the very thing that ends the overtrainer's cycle and maybe even her workout career. Body-building guru Joe Weider used to tell Robert that the only thing that makes many people stop doing crazy workouts or training too hard or doing too much for too long is their bodies finally saying, "Enough! Here's an injury for you and that'll make you stop."

But, we have a better solution.

Forced rest breaks in your strength-training routine.

Years ago, the old-school athletes didn't have access to the scientific research and understanding about elite athletes that we have today. They simply had to rely on what their bodies were telling them (*still* great advice for everyone!). They became very sensitive to the feedback their bodies gave them. How did they look and feel? How were their strength and recovery? Were they progressing? How quickly or slowly were the results coming? There were many other "feedback markers" they set up and constantly monitored inside and outside of the gym.

Having an injury was a cardinal sin of training that told them and others, with few exceptions, that they had been careless and foolish. An injured athlete hadn't listened to his or her body and what it was saying.

Then the wisest among them began experimenting with the concept of taking regular rest breaks. That is, even if they were making great progress, they purposely stopped training for a limited period of time, then returned to training at a pace and intensity below where their last training cycle had ended—some of them well below that level.

But here's what it accomplished for them.

- They stopped while their bodies were still making great progress.

- They stopped before any injuries or overtraining symptoms showed up.

- They began the next training cycle with even greater energy, ability, and capacity to generate power and enhanced recuperative ability.

In my years of training and working with numerous people all over the world, I've found that a good training/rest cycle for many people is 1 complete week off (with zero training) for every 4 to 6 weeks of working out. Then, when you're ready to start the next 4- to

6-week training cycle, begin your workouts at least 30 percent below the level at which you ended your last training cycle. For example, if you could do a dumbbell biceps curl with a 15-pound dumbbell in each hand for 8 reps at the time you took your forced rest break, then you'd begin your new training cycle using 30 percent less weight, which would be with a 10-pound dumbbell in each hand.

Experiment with this to find the ideal training/rest cycle that will keep you injury-free and on the road to lifelong results.

Menopause Reset! Testimonials

From Patients . . .

I've been a patient of Dr. Mickey's, off and on, for over 10 years. It has been one of the most rewarding relationships of my life. His enthusiasm for living well is contagious and the passion he has for his craft is infectious. What I found to be of greater value than his abundant knowledge of human nutrition and fitness is his phenomenal ability to motivate me to be better, to be grander. Not only would I have never completed a marathon without his guidance, but I never would have believed in my abilities enough to attempt such a feat. Dr. Mickey has the most remarkable, and genuine, ability to dare you to believe in all that you are capable of and then provide you with the tools to get there.

Ten years later, I am still learning from him; each office visit surprises me with new knowledge and continued support. I prefer not to imagine how different my life would be had I not made the first appointment with Dr. Mickey. Being in the best shape of my life and preparing for another marathon is somewhere I never dreamed I would be at 38 years old. Dr. Mickey's love of life and ability to educate and encourage is sincere and heartfelt, and quite difficult to articulate. I am eternally grateful for all the things he has taught me, the optimal health he has enabled me to obtain and for encouraging me to believe beyond my own limitations.

—*Jill Roese, CT*

I am a patient/friend of Dr. Mickey Harpaz. I am a diabetic and a heart patient. When I was last in Connecticut, my sugar level was between 200 to 300 range (quite high), and my internist increased my meds. Dr. Mick put me on a very easy program of diet and exercise. I was to eat every 2 hours (mostly fruits in between meals) and try to exercise at least 10 minutes in the a.m. and 10 minutes in the p.m.

The eating every 2 hours is sometimes a chore, as I feel "full" some of the times. The exercising can be a problem as I have other health issues (arthritic knees, bad back, etc.). I'm up to 30 minutes on the treadmill when I can. All in all, I feel that I'm achieving a lot of results.

So far, I've lost 16 pounds. My sugar levels have also dropped considerably—92 at lunchtime yesterday to usually in the 120 range. I am still on diabetic meds, but hopefully soon, when it is regulated more, I will be able to eliminate them.

I live in South Florida, and right now, even indoors, it is difficult to exercise. Working out in this oppressive heat is very hard. I'm trying my best.

I thank Dr. Mick for all of his help and getting me on the right track to take control of my health.

—*Enid Hurwitz, FL*

I'm a 55-year-old woman, and I have an angel on my shoulder. His name is Dr. Mickey Harpaz, and I'm so grateful that he resides there. Every 2 hours I feel his gentle caring presence, and I am reminded to eat a piece of fruit, some veggies, perhaps some yogurt.

About a year ago, an orthopedist informed me that my bone density was diminishing at a rapid pace and that immediate action was necessary to ward off osteoporosis. His instructions were: "Here, take this prescription to your pharmacist and call me in a year." . . . Thanks very much.

Not one to take pharmaceuticals lightly, I wanted an alternative. The answer was not hard to find.

My husband, who was diagnosed with type 2 diabetes, was already under Dr. Mick's care. Within 1 year, he had lost 50 pounds and his diabetes is now under control with drugs, healthy eating, and daily exercise.

I needed a personalized, informative approach to treating my osteopenia. So, I now also work with Dr. Mick, who patiently waits while I take notes, makes certain that I understand the dynamics of eating every 2 hours, that I supplement my diet with calcium and why I *must* make time (30 minutes each day) for myself—not for anyone else—just for me. *And*, that's my medicine for maintaining healthy bones.

It's not difficult to understand or to pull off. And Dr. Mick truly and deeply cares about my success!

So off I go, to take my magic pill: a bunch of pushups, a 30-minute walk through the woods, and some calcium . . . not bad.

Thank you, Dr. Mick.

—Laurie, Danbury, CT

I have experienced the most positive life-altering changes after working with Mickey over the past 4 years.

I sought out Dr. Harpaz at a time when I felt I had run out of options. I had gained weight following the death of my mother and had tried to lose the weight without success.

Mickey was immediately positive and supportive and set me on the course to success. His individualized attention, simple-to-follow plan, and unwavering positive attitude kept me focused and led me to where I am today. I have dropped two dress sizes and lost a huge amount of body fat. I exercise 7 days a week where I used to exercise three or four times a week. I am mindful of what I eat, but never feel deprived or like I'm on a diet. I feel better, look better, and am in the best physical shape I've ever been.

Mickey is one of the most inspirational and motivational people I've had the pleasure of knowing, and he has changed the way I live my life.

—Kathy Klotz, CT

After a decade of yo-yo dieting and an obsession with the scale, I met Dr. Mickey Harpaz, and my life changed. It was 6 months before my wedding, and I was in a state of panic because my dress didn't fit.

I had spent years hiding from the camera and wanted this celebration to be different. On the day of our meeting, I agreed to throw out my scale and say good-bye to my addiction to fad diets. I committed myself to Mickey's approach to eating. At first, I was terrified to let go of "dieting" and daily weigh-ins, but I was feeling desperate, and this was my last-ditch effort. The wedding photos and relaxed smile on my face say everything about the success of Mickey's help.

That was 12 years ago, and I have easily maintained my figure through three pregnancies and a series of other life-changing events. I do not own a scale, and I never "diet." Mickey taught me how to think about nutrition and exercise in a way that makes sense as a way of life.

—Sara Wheeler, CT

"No matter what I do, I can't lose any weight. . . . "

That was my first conversation with Dr. Mickey, in a nutshell. When I first met him, something was missing in my daily routine. I was working really hard, with minimal results, and I had an obsession with the number on the scale. We are led to believe that with proper diet and exercise, weight loss is close behind. But that wasn't true for me. The last straw was after I'd competed in a 6-week fitness challenge, which included hours in the gym every day and three spin classes a week, nothing changed. I was ecstatic to finish second overall, but there was no weight loss and no change to my BMI, measured at the start.

I was introduced to Dr. Mickey Harpaz through a mutual friend. In just a week, he adjusted not so much what I ate, but when I ate. The adjustment to eating on a more consistent schedule, as well as continuing my daily workout routine was the absolute missing piece to the puzzle! I was amazed to see results in just 2 weeks. With visible results, I was determined to give 110 percent to Mickey's program. I could not stay off of the scale initially, but now I have learned that the scale doesn't always tell the real story, and it is just a number.

Fast forward 9 months, and not only have I surpassed my initial goal, but I have lost 18 percent body fat (currently at 14.7 percent). Together with Mickey's encouragement and my own inner desire to challenge myself, I chose a goal that seemed attainable, but certainly not easy: I am now training for my first 5-K run in September. I never thought I could run 5 minutes, much less 5 miles, but now I have a new tool to choose for my workout regimen. I have to say that at 42 years old, I am in the best shape of my life thanks to Dr. Mickey!

—*Carolyn Reed, CT*

When I gave Mickey a call last May, it was an act of desperation. Over the past 2 years, I had gained about 15 pounds and was unable to lose them. I was so depressed that I cried every day. It wasn't that 15 pounds was so awful, but more that I couldn't stop gaining and I didn't see an end in sight!

As a menopausal woman of 54, nothing was working for me. I worked out twice a week with a trainer, did my cardio, and tried to watch what I ate. As the pounds crept on, I sought advice from everyone and everywhere.

The magazines and books said, "No carbs." My trainer recommended more intense workouts and interval training. Others talked about more soy, more protein, less fruit, and no alcohol! (Wait a minute—I am in menopause . . . I need a glass of wine now and then!) I tried them all, and nothing worked for me. I just kept slowly gaining, and the rolls around my middle just kept growing.

When I walked into Mickey's office, he asked me what I wanted, and I told him I just wanted my body back! He gave me a plan that was so doable and so simple that I was thrilled. I immediately felt like the weight of the world had been lifted from my shoulders.

Using his plan, I walked daily and ate every 2 hours. The wonderful thing is that I wasn't ever hungry and I completely lost my cravings for sweets. Amazing! What a relief to not have to frantically search for the next diet craze.

In 6 months I dropped 10 pounds and went from 38 percent body fat to 19 percent body fat! Everyone wants to know my secret.

The wonderful thing is that it is easy and there are no gimmicks. I eat regular food, feel great, and can do this plan forever!

—*Mary Swett, CT*

It is very definitely a partnership when you work with Dr. Harpaz. It's as though he is a companion on your journey as you make these changes in lifestyle: daily exercise and proper nutrition.

Everything is presented in a straightforward and methodical manner. He makes it as easy as possible to follow the prescribed regimen for bringing blood sugar under control.

—*Ms. Pat Kelly, CT*

I am a 58-year-old woman with a family history of diabetes. My mother and both of her parents were diabetic. My mother and grandmother lost a leg to this dreadful disease. Needless to say, I was panic struck when I was told that my blood sugar was 160.

I immediately contacted Dr. Harpaz and begged him to help me. I told him that I would do anything to avoid the nightmare that my mom endured. He assured me that although my family background was a strong factor in my elevated sugar, I was not predestined to my mom's fate. He told me that if I ate at regular intervals, and in small quantities, my sugar would gradually return to normal.

I was determined to reach this goal. Within 1 week my sugar levels started to slowly decline. Within 1 month they were well on their way to within normal ranges. Within 6 weeks they were below 100, and I lost 40 pounds!

I can't thank Dr. Harpaz enough for helping me. Today I am still controlling my sugar levels, and I am not on any medication. I owe this miracle to Dr. Harpaz.

—*Mrs. W., Sonshine, CT*

Dr. Mickey Harpaz has done wonderful things for our family. My late husband suffered many problems because of his heart, and he loved food. Dr. Harpaz worked with him over the years through nutritional consultation to reduce his weight and give him more years of life.

I have personally recommended Dr. Harpaz to a number of people, because besides his regular consulting, he has become a friend and he shows great interest in understanding the whole person. He gives you tips and ideas on how to satisfy cravings and how much exercise and what kind you need to stay in good condition. He has meant so much to my family.

—*Mrs. D., Jackson, CT*

Dear Dr. Harpaz,
I can tell you truthfully, no matter what exercise I do, the principles of healthy eating that you taught me have remained a part of my life no matter what. I talk about your program often and thank you for trying to reach the rest of the world.

Not only has nutrition and exercise become a passion for me, I am currently helping to bring the "Just Run" program of California into our schools here in my area. These values and the values you taught me about food will forever be a part of my life. You are an amazing doctor and educator. I hope you never give up!

Peace and happiness to you and all of your family.

—*Karen U., New Hope, PA*

When I first found out that I was expecting, I was very excited, but I was also determined to be somewhat in control of my changing body. I started Dr. Harpaz's program when I was 10 weeks into my pregnancy, and since then I have continued to lose body fat, although I have gained weight because of my growing baby.

My daily exercise along with my newly acquired dietary habits have helped me not only because it is important to stay active but also because it has eliminated some "side effects" of being pregnant like heartburn, swelling, and constipation.

The best part of the program for me is that I have been able to control my gestational diabetes without any insulin and virtually any efforts.

Following the program has been easier because of Dr. Harpaz's approach: He educated me instead of just giving me strict rules to follow.

Now at the end of my pregnancy, I am happy to say that I have been able to reach my goal of controlling my changing body, thanks to Dr. Harpaz's guidance and support.

—*Claudia Giuliani, CT*

I was diagnosed with type 1 diabetes about 3 years ago. At first, controlling my diabetes was manageable. After I had my first child, my sugar levels began to spiral out of control, plus I was unable to lose my pregnancy weight. The Dr. Harpaz Plan enabled me to control my sugars and helped to begin the post-pregnancy weight loss.

I am now pregnant with my second child. About 3 months into my pregnancy my sugar levels started hitting dangerous lows (30s) and highs above 250. I immediately scheduled an appointment to begin getting the sugar levels and my anxiety under control. After several weeks of working on my meal plans, timing of meals, and exercise routine, I have been able to stabilize my sugar levels and my anxiety. Plus, after gaining 40 pounds during my first pregnancy, I have been able to keep my weight gain to a little over 16 pounds by month 7.

—*Mrs. L. Fuccillo, CT*

From Doctors . . .

I first met Mickey when he came to speak to my office about nutrition, healthy eating, and weight loss. He spoke about how I could help guide my patients in healthy eating and exercise. Soon after we met, I decided to make an appointment with him so that he could help me lose the 10 extra pounds that I'd been trying to lose over the last few years. Since becoming his patient, I have learned to eat well, eat healthy, and excrcise properly. I have learned to read food labels and to maintain an overall healthy lifestyle. Since I joined his program, I have felt lighter, healthier, and more energized. He is an expert at what he does, he is motivating, and he really wants you to succeed. My experience with him has been wonderful, and I have implemented his guidance in my life. I give out his advice to my patients. My experience with him has been great, and I would recommend him to anyone!

—*Maryam Hedayatzadeh, MD, CT*

Dr. Mickey Harpaz combines a solid knowledge of exercise physiology and nutrition with good common sense and lots of enthusiasm. His individualized "healthy heart" programs have helped a large number of my patients with problems ranging from diabetes, premenopausal and menopausal, high blood pressure, coronary artery disease, high cholesterol to simple obesity.

His one-on-one and group sessions teach patients the fundamentals of a healthy lifestyle, while his dynamic personality motivates them to convert principles into practice. Dr. Harpaz has often succeeded where other diet and exercise programs have failed.

—*Carolyn Becker, MD, FACP*

We realize today that weight reduction involves a commitment to a change in lifestyle, a lifestyle with good diet and carefully planned exercise program.

Over the past few years we have referred a large number of our patients to Dr. Harpaz and have been very pleased with his program of diet and exercise retraining, leading to long-term results, not the "quick fix" so common today.

—*Jay Weiner, MD*

I have known Dr. Mickey Harpaz for 15 years. I have the highest regard for his abilities in helping my patients reduce their weight, blood pressure, and cholesterol and control diabetes through a system of sound nutritional advice as well as his infectious enthusiasm for exercise.

I must say that whenever I have patients who are sedentary, I strongly encourage them to see Dr. Harpaz. Somehow he manages to get them motivated to exercise and to achieve a healthy lifestyle.

—*Jeffrey S. Metzger, MD*

I have known personally and professionally Dr. Mickey Harpaz for the last 8 years. Dr. Harpaz is a skilled nutritionist as well as an exercise physiologist who works well in helping patients achieve and maintain healthy diet and exercise lifestyles. We co-managed many patients over the years, and I have sought his expertise for my own personal wellness and for that of my family.

—*Patrice S. Gillotti, MD*

Special Report by Dr. Harpaz and Mr. Wolff

Get Your Body Back with the Sweet 16

IT'S TIME TO MAKE THE BODY YOU HAVE INTO THE BODY YOU'VE ALWAYS WANTED

While we may never have met you, we have something that we know you want.

How do we know?

Because we know you haven't been happy with the way you look and feel.

You're sick and tired of trying diet after diet, reading book after book and magazine after magazine, and buying gadget after gadget, and all you have to show for it is money wasted and a body that's tired and out of shape and has little or no energy.

You've felt like giving up.

You've felt like it's no use.

And you've felt like there's no hope.

But you've been wrong!

What we're about to share with you is something we like to call the Sweet 16.

Why do we call it the Sweet 16?

Because it's a collection of 16 tips that are so simple that most of the women who look and feel great have used them for years and don't even realize it.

Here's how we discovered them.

One day while we were talking about our travels to many places throughout the world, we began talking about what we had observed women of all ages do to stay leaner and healthier.

As we began comparing notes, it dawned on us that we could identify 16 very specific approaches—from thinking to diet to exercise—these women were using to help them either lose weight or prevent it from ever being a problem in their lives.

You see, the most powerful way to change how you look and feel doesn't come from a pill, exercise machine, or video.

You don't need to join an expensive health club, exercise for hours, eat like a bird, or even eat foods you don't like. For years, you may have done that—and look where it's gotten you.

It's time to stop.

No, friend, looking and feeling your best is not something reserved for the chosen lucky few. You see, one of the easiest, quickest, and most effective ways for you to change how you look and feel—and sustain the change—is to use the tips in this book. If you want an extra boost of power to keep you on the right road to diet and fitness success, then also follow our Sweet 16 tips.

Once you do, here's what you can expect.

- A leaner, firmer body

- More energy than you've had in years

- Looser-fitting clothes (we hope you won't mind buying a brand-new, smaller-size wardrobe)

- A lower stress level and a happier attitude

- Deeper sleep, more relaxation, and better rest

- Better digestion

- Reduced chances of injury and disease

- Improved self-esteem and a positive self-image

- More confidence

- More success

- And much, much more!

If you want to have more energy; a leaner, stronger, and firmer body; a healthier body; a shapelier body; and a better-looking body, then the Sweet 16 could be just what you've been looking for.

If you apply the Sweet 16 tips in your life and do the simple and easy things we're about to share with you, we know you'll be inspired and happy with the results you're about to experience. And it'll help you stay motivated to get the body you want. (You can admit it: staying motivated has been a problem, right?)

We created the Sweet 16 to be a simple step-by-step guide, and it is proven to help menopausal women take back control of their bodies and self-images. And, it will help you look and feel better than you may ever have imagined was possible.

When that happens, and it will, you'll be enjoying life again—perhaps like you never have before. And knowing that we've helped you change your life and the way you look and feel is the greatest reward we could ever ask for.

Before we give you the Sweet 16, you might be asking yourself how those 16 tips can be so different from everything else you've tried that they'll make the difference this time.

Good question.

Because the Sweet 16 tips are based on simple principles that have not and will not change—that is, unless they build a new version of the human body.

Don't worry; they won't.

These principles have been around for many years. Sure, foods change. Exercise equipment changes. And so do all those diet books and videos, but principles—make that *these principles*—do not.

We think you're going to be amazed by how easy they'll be to use.

By using the strategies and advice you've been reading in the book in combination with these tips, you'll have the power to direct your body to look and feel its best because you're the one who decides just how good you want to look and feel and how quickly you want it to happen.

So here's how to use these tips.

Use a few of the Sweet 16 tips if you want good results, and use more of the tips anytime you want *better* results. The choice is always up to you.

Always remember that it doesn't take much effort or giant life changes to make a big difference in how you look and feel.

Not hour after hour of exercise.

Not radical dieting or changes in eating.

Not cupboards full of supplements.

Not expensive equipment or health club memberships.

And not jumping on the latest diet or fitness trend.

It takes making simple steps: simple steps that we have observed over our years of travel and working with women just like you, steps that are easy to understand and to include in your life and will be enjoyable for you.

The women who experience and enjoy the longest-lasting diet and fitness success are those who make these tips daily parts of their lives. In only a short time, following these tips became automatic for these women, and they are now such a part of their daily lives that they rarely, if ever, think about them.

The same is about to happen for you.

Enjoy!

SWEET 16 TIP #1—MAKE A NEW PICTURE

Women who lose weight or stay at the same great-looking and great-feeling weight for years and years have accepted in their minds a specific picture of how they should look and feel. This picture is so clear and vivid that anything else simply would be unacceptable.

They see and know what it feels like to always be able to slip into their favorite jeans, skirts, pants, and dresses. They see and know what it feels like to always buy the same size of underwear and lingerie. They see and know what it feels like to go to the store and buy the same-size tops and know that they will fit.

And they know these things because the pictures they keep playing in their minds reinforce and support their eating and exercise habits, which, in turn, keep them doing just the right amounts of activities and eating the right amounts and kinds of foods to keep their pictures of themselves a reality day after day, week after week, and year after year.

Tip #1 Take-Away:
Create a new picture of how you want to look.

SWEET 16 TIP #2—SAY DIFFERENT WORDS

Women with great-looking bodies speak to themselves in different ways than women who see themselves as fat, out of shape, and needing to lose weight do.

And though they may not realize it, women who look and feel great understand a powerful truth: *You can't have a 130-pound body if you keep thinking like a 160-pound person.*

Women with healthy and nice-looking bodies think differently. For one, they don't tell themselves that they're fat or that they need to lose weight. Such negative words and thoughts give the brain a very powerful message, and that is "Fat . . . fat . . . fat . . . you're fat!"

And what does the brain do with such a message? It brings things into your life that agree with the kinds of thoughts, words, beliefs, and pictures you're giving it. If these messages to yourself are about how out of shape, heavy, flabby, or fat you are, then the message the brain hears and responds to is, "Stay fat," which keeps you just the way you keep telling yourself you don't want to be!

The truth is, society may be obsessed with how women look or should look, but the majority of women with consistently healthy and nice-looking bodies actually think very little about their bodies. The images they have in their minds, which they accepted years before, are the only ones they accept, and there's no need to keep thinking about them since they keep giving them results they're very happy with.

Tip #2 Take-Away:
Keep your thoughts, words, and beliefs on the things you want and let go of the things you don't.

SWEET 16 TIP #3—EAT THE RIGHT FOODS

Women with healthy and good-looking bodies watch what they eat, but they are not fanatical. They're not obsessed with how much carbohydrates, protein, and fat they eat. They know that the importance lies not so much in the *kinds* of calories they eat as in how *many* calories they eat.

If they eat more than their bodies can use, they put on weight; if they eat fewer calories than they need, they'll lose weight. But none of that is a worry to them since their mental pictures—the images they've accepted of how they should look and feel—always keep them within a few pounds of their ideal weight, year after year.

They eat small meals every few hours throughout the day and rarely miss breakfast. They eat a wide variety of foods. They'll have sweets, breads, cookies, and all other kinds of snacks, but they do so rarely, and when they do, they don't eat much of them.

They give their bodies what they crave whenever they crave it, but they just won't eat a lot of it. They know that when we forcibly keep ourselves away from the things we love, it only makes us think about and want them that much more. And when we do finally get them, we overindulge and eat too much.

Yet, when they allow themselves to eat what they want when they want, then the powerful craving goes away and they actually end up eating very little of their treat since they know they can have it again at any time they desire. The end result is that they eat much less.

Women who have lost weight and kept it off eat very little processed foods and will choose to eat a variety of vegetables, some fruits (though not a lot), and lots of different sources of protein, and, once the weight is off, they can even use things like real butter (not margarine), real sour cream (not just fat-free), and whole eggs (not just egg whites).

Women with healthy and good-looking bodies aren't affected by carbohydrate cravings like other women. These women have more fats and protein and less carbohydrates in their diet and because of it, their insulin, blood sugar, and energy levels are very consistent throughout the day, without the ups and downs that eating too many carbohydrates or not enough calories can bring.

Because women with terrific bodies have more fats (the good fats) and proteins (always remember that if it swims, flies, grazes, or has beans, nuts, or soy, think of it as a good protein food for you to eat) in their diets, they don't get hungry as often.

And even though every 2 or so hours they'll eat breakfast, lunch, dinner, or a snack, they eat smaller portions—which helps their bodies more efficiently assimilate the foods they eat—and their total calorie intake for the day is actually *lower* than that of the women who miss meals, eat junk foods for snacks, and have larger portions when they do eat meals.

Tip #3 Take-Away:
Eat what you want when you want, don't eat a lot of it, and choose from a wide variety of foods.

SWEET 16 TIP #4—HAVE SMALLER PORTIONS

Women who are healthy and at their ideal weight know they can have the healthiest diet imaginable, but if they eat too many calories and more nutrients than their bodies need, they'll gain weight.

Their secret is to eat whatever they want whenever they want it, but to eat smaller portions.

The body can use smaller portions of foods better than it can if it only gets one or two large meals in a day.

Think of your body using food like you working on your list of things to do. If you have only a few tasks to complete, then it's much easier for you to take the time, devote the right amount of energy, and focus on doing each of those tasks well. And that's the way the body works when it's fed smaller portions of good foods at each meal. It makes better use of the food it's being fed.

However, if you have not one, two, three, or four things to do at once but many, it's easy to become overwhelmed, lose focus and concentration, and become far less effective at getting each of those many tasks completed.

The body is the same way when you feed it only one or two big meals that have more food and nutrients than it can effectively use. The result is that fewer nutrients get used, more get wasted, and more get stored as excess calories or fat.

Tip #4 Take-Away:
Think small—as in smaller portions—and eat smaller meals more frequently throughout the day.

Sweet 16 Tip #5—Use Smaller Cups, Plates, Bowls, and Utensils

Women who stay the same size year after year do a few things other women don't, and one of them is using smaller cooking and eating utensils. There can be many reasons why. Some may have learned it from their mothers or grandmothers. Others may have limited space in the smaller living areas that are more common in Asia than in Western countries, so they had to buy smaller plates, bowls, cups, spoons, and forks. Yet, both of these reasons had—and continue to have—a very powerful influence on keeping them leaner, healthier, and looking and weighing the same.

Using smaller cups, plates, and bowls means that smaller portions are consumed each time you eat or drink—and that means fewer calories. Using smaller bowls could cut the amount you eat in half compared to the portion held by a regular-size bowl in the United States.

Smaller utensils mean you can only eat small portions each time you use that utensil. You take smaller bites, you take more of those bites, and your meals therefore take longer to eat, giving your brain time to receive signals from your stomach that you have had enough food. This is the very thing that women miss out on when they eat too much too quickly.

Another thing you can do is to use chopsticks. If you've ever seen or used chopsticks, you know that you can't hold too much food with them and that it takes many passes with the chopsticks to eat your meal—and therefore more time to eat that meal, which gives your brain time to tell you you've had enough.

And it does one other thing: It allows your brain time to speak to you and tell you some powerful messages that include:

- "You've already eaten one bowl of food . . ." (even if it is a smaller bowl, the brain only thinks of it as one bowl of food) ". . . and you don't need any more."

- "You've been eating for a long time now . . ." (smaller utensils and bowls and plates force you to take longer to eat) ". . . and it's time to quit."

Tip #5 Take-Away:
Use smaller bowls, plates, and utensils for big results.

SWEET 16 TIP #6—EAT SLOWLY

There's an old European spa secret that women who visit them have used for years: eat slowly, chew slowly, and chew often.

One of the problems overweight women in Western countries face is eating too much too quickly, without properly chewing their food—which is one of the most important steps in digestion.

The European women have it right.

For one, they eat slowly. Not only does this allow them to enjoy and savor the foods they eat—in Europe, a meal is an event that is not to be rushed—it also allows their bodies to tell them when to stop eating when they have had enough food.

They also chew each mouthful 10 to 20 times before it is swallowed. This helps break down the food and release its nutrients much more efficiently and makes it easier for the stomach, digestive juices, and other organs to do their jobs more quickly and better. These women report that they feel they have better digestion, more effectively use the foods they've eaten, and have less bloating and water retention. Try it and you'll see why it is so highly recommended.

Tip #6 Take-Away:
Eat more slowly and chew for longer.

Sweet 16 Tip #7—Eat and Drink Hot and Cold

Here's another simple thing that women without weight problems do: They eat and drink hot and cold beverages and foods.

Wonder why?

Besides enjoying them, doing so has beneficial effects on their metabolisms and appetites.

For example, women have told us that hot and spicy foods make them sweat (don't worry, it's a good thing) and that they can really feel a difference throughout their bodies—they feel like their metabolisms are more active. If you've ever bitten into a jalapeño chile pepper, you know what they're talking about! But you don't have to go that far to get the effects of eating foods that are hot and spicy (to a level you're comfortable with).

The other thing they do is drink hot and cold liquids.

From ice water and iced tea to hot coffee and hot tea, drinking hot and cold beverages makes your body burn more calories than it would if you drank room-temperature or slightly cooled or heated fluids.

The body uses extra calories to heat cold drinks to the temperature the body needs them at in order to process them. Similarly, the body uses extra calories to cool hot drinks to the temperature the body needs them at to process them.

The same thing happens for higher temperature and spicy foods, because any food that is too hot must be cooled down to the body's acceptable range of temperatures for using, processing, and digesting that food.

All of these things make the body use more calories, and those extra calories can mean the difference between a body that stays overweight and one that begins to slowly shed pounds.

Tip #7 Take-Away:
Be hot, be cold, and be spicy.

SWEET 16 TIP #8—EAT ON TIME

Women with healthy bodies eat on time and rarely miss meals or deviate from this schedule.

Eating at regular times during the day keeps their energy and blood sugar levels stable, helps prevent hunger urges and binges, and greatly reduces carbohydrate cravings for sweets and other foods with non-nutritious and excess fat-producing calories.

These women know firsthand how well their bodies respond to being fed and hydrated throughout the day. They also know that when the body gets the nutrients it needs when it needs them, it operates very smoothly. And when the body is satisfied, so is the brain, making thoughts of how they look and feel or how hungry they are and other food issues arise rarely since they look and feel great the majority of the time.

Breakfast is the most important meal of the day for them, and it is usually a meal with lots of protein, some fats, and carbohydrates— perhaps a small glass of fresh juice or a piece of fruit.

And they do something else: They cascade their eating from the first meal until the last meal at night. That is, they eat the larger meals (especially those high in carbohydrates) earlier in the day, decreasing their carbohydrate intake and the sizes of their meals as the day goes on. Breakfast is the biggest meal, lunch is the same size or smaller than breakfast, and dinner is smaller than lunch.

They also have small, nutritious snacks (with protein sources like tofu, a piece of cheese or cottage cheese, or fresh vegetables like celery, carrots, or broccoli)—if they desire—every 2 hours between breakfast and dinner and a high-protein snack (like cottage cheese with pineapple or strawberries) 90 minutes or so before bedtime.

These women also eat slightly bigger meals than normal prior to doing any kind of activity that demands more energy. This could be exercising, working in the yard or garden, doing chores in the house, working extra-hard at work, or performing lots of errands. This is just the opposite of what many women do; instead, they have a big meal at the end of the day or after finishing the activity.

The key is to give the body the extra fuel and nutrients it needs *prior* to the activity, not after. That way, it will use those extra calories more efficiently.

Tip #8 Take-Away:
Eat on time and at the right times.

SWEET 16 TIP #9—EAT A VARIETY OF FOODS

Variety is the spice (and enjoyment) of eating and life, and women who have terrific bodies eat lots of different foods.

Far too many women who don't have great bodies make the mistake of eating too much of only a few kinds of foods and not eating enough of others, and as a result, their bodies might develop an intolerance and sometimes even allergies to some of those foods.

Eating too much of one kind of food can also prevent the body from effectively assimilating and using the nutrients from that food. Nutrients that normally would be used efficiently if they were eaten only in moderation may be excreted unused or more easily processed for fat storage.

The women who have healthy, beautiful bodies are not big junk food eaters. Desire for these carbohydrates typically comes from not having enough protein and fats in the diet or, as you read earlier in the book, not eating small meals frequently. When they do rarely have junk food, they have it in small amounts, which keeps it from negatively affecting how they look and feel.

Tip # 9 Take-Away:
Eat many different kinds of foods.

SWEET 16 TIP #10—THE ANSWER IS CLEAR: DRINK WATER, AND LOTS OF IT

Women with great-looking, healthy bodies drink plenty of water. They drink it throughout the day—not just a few times a day when they think about it or get thirsty—and they drink lots of it.

Despite the latest research that says you may not need the often-recommended eight glasses of water a day, these women have found that thirst is not the best signal for when it's time to drink water. By the time the brain receives the signal that the body is thirsty, it's already too late; the body will have needed some water for quite some time.

The smart women are those who have small drinks and sips throughout their day. And yes, they do go to the restroom more frequently, though not that much more, and whenever they go there, they receive an important message: If the urine is clear, their bodies are getting enough water.

And whether these women know it or not, there are also some huge benefits from drinking lots of water. They are:

1. Since their bodies are hydrated (well-watered) on the inside, their skin is hydrated on the outside. They have less dry skin.

2. Water helps mobilize and use fatty acids, which helps their bodies more efficiently burn fat for fuel.

3. Muscles need water, and muscles are needed to perform any activity or do any job. If the body doesn't get enough water, the muscles are negatively affected, leading to poor performance. But when the body gets enough water, the muscles work much more effectively, for better results.

Perhaps one of the biggest surprises women with great bodies have discovered is that when they give their bodies all the water they need, they don't retain water or bloat.

And there's a good reason why.

Women with out-of-shape bodies make the mistake of believing that they should reduce their water intake if they want to lose weight.

So, they reduce it and not much happens.

They reduce it some more and then they begin to feel bloated.

They reduce it even more and their bodies do just the opposite of what they thought they would; they feel more bloated than before they started this whole mess.

They don't realize why their bodies are doing what they are doing.

You see, if the body doesn't get the water it needs when it needs it, it holds on to whatever water it does have or gets because it doesn't know when it's going to get more water. Remember what you read about triggering the body's self-defense mechanism against starvation when you don't give it enough food or feed it often enough?

Not giving your body enough water triggers a sort of starvation response: It holds on to what you have because it doesn't know when more is coming. The body wants to preserve itself, and it does so by slowing down the metabolism and holding on to fluid.

But if you're like the smart, healthy women with great bodies and you do what they do—give your body all the water it needs through-out the day—then just the opposite happens.

The body releases the fluids it was holding on to because it now knows it's getting water—and lots of it—and there's no need to hold on to any excess fluids. End result: The body is healthier and performs and looks so much better.

Tip #10 Take-Away:
Keep your body watered throughout the day.

Sweet 16 Tip #11—Be Active

If you want to have a great-looking body, then you need to do what the women who have lean bodies do, and that is be active.

It's all about moving your body.

But you don't need hours of aerobics, long sweaty workouts, personal trainers, expensive health club memberships, new workout clothes, or supplements to do it.

The key thing to remember is that small activities pay off in big results for toning your body or burning extra calories.

Women who look and feel great are not obsessed with how many minutes they're on a stairclimber or treadmill. They keep themselves busy, whether it's at work, home, or school. They do lots of little activities that, when added up at the end of the day, total more energy burned and muscles used than you may ever have imagined possible.

These women have regular lives—just like you—and most of them don't have a 30-, 40-, or 60-minute block of time in their day to devote to just working out.

But they don't need it, since the results from exercise and being active are cumulative—they all add up.

That means that 5 minutes of activity here in the morning, 10 minutes of activity there in the afternoon, and 15 minutes of being busy at night add up to 30 minutes of muscles exercised and calories burned without any extra thought or effort. All by simply doing the things they do during the day.

And these women will tell you that the most important thing that helps them stay lean is being active.

- Move your legs.

- Move your arms.

- Move your body.

- Don't sit so much.

- Take longer strides when you walk.

- Walk a little bit faster.

- Walk for a little bit longer.

- Park farther away than you normally would.

- Carry heavier bags of groceries.

- Walk up and down more steps by taking the stairs instead of the elevator.

Just do the things you do in your normal daily living with just a little extra effort and you'll be amazed by the results.

Tip #11 Take-Away:
Be active and keep your body moving.

SWEET 16 TIP #12—GET PLENTY OF REST

Women who have healthy, nice-looking bodies get plenty of rest.

They go to bed at nearly the same time every night and wake up at nearly the same time every morning. Almost like clockwork, these women easily fall asleep because they used their active bodies during the day and kept their thoughts positive, happy, calm, and relaxed. They wake up ready for another great day and all the possibilities it can bring.

Sure, there are days when the stresses of work, school, family, friends, and relationships keep them awake longer than usual, but those times are few.

Yes, there are times when they do too much physical or mental activity during the day, but those times are rare.

And there are times when they break with their normal daily schedule by working or staying out late, traveling on business, or going on vacation, but they are the exceptions in an otherwise pre-dictable schedule.

Just like food and water, the body thrives on regular periods of rest and sleep. Many of these women have found the ideal amount of sleep to be anywhere from 7 to 9 hours each night. Some like a little more, and others prefer a little less. Others, especially those with kids to raise, may not get a solid 6 to 8 hours a night, but they have micro-naps (periods of rest that last for 5 to 15 minutes) at various times throughout the day.

Your body needs sleep and rest to recuperate, repair, and rejuvenate itself so it can keep your body, heart, and soul operating at their best the next day.

Give your body the rest it needs, and the rest will take care of itself.

Tip #12 Take-Away:
Be well rested to look and feel great.

SWEET 16 TIP #13—ALWAYS HAVE THINGS TO DO

There's a maxim about being happy in one's life that says, "Life is exciting in proportion to the number of things you have to look forward to."

Having few things to look forward to equals little excitement.

Having many things to look forward to equals much excitement.

Women who look and feel great invariably have many things they want to accomplish, be they as simple as working in the garden, running errands with the kids, making sure the family is looked after, studying a new subject, or working on an important project.

Women with many things to do and look forward to are those who love to stay busy. They're masters at accomplishing goals—often by accomplishing lots of smaller goals that, when added up, equal a very big goal.

And when they're working on their goals, they're staying busy—thinking, being, doing, becoming—and when they're busy, they're active. Activity uses the mind and the body's muscles, and it also uses calories—extra calories that would likely become extra pounds for those who aren't as busy or who don't have things to look forward to.

The wonderful thing about being busy for women who look and feel great is that they are the ones who decide just how busy they want to be.

They are the ones who create and determine the things they want to look forward to.

They are the ones who set the goals, accomplish the goals, and feel the rewards.

And they are the ones who, by doing these things, make their minds, bodies, and spirits things to feel really good about.

Tip #13 Take-Away:
Having things to look forward to can change your mind,
your body, and your life.

SWEET 16 TIP #14—THROW AWAY THE SCALE

One thing you may find at the home of a woman with a great body is a bathroom scale. However, *rarely* will it be used.

Many women who have kept the same healthy and lean body go through their lives without ever seeing a scale or knowing about the damage it can do to a woman who lives by its numbers.

Others—typically in Western countries—who have experienced firsthand the powerful forces of persuasion and judgment the media and culture exert upon women and the negative effects they can have on self-image and self-esteem have decided to say no to the scale and yes to being kinder to themselves and treating themselves better. They treat themselves just like a best friend would, who likes you not for how you look, but for *who you are* inside.

Women with great bodies know that the scale simply tells a number that does not, and cannot, tell them how good they look or how terrific they feel.

Yet, for those who don't have a strong self-esteem or a body they're happy with, the scale only adds to their frustration. Though it displays a neutral number (neither good nor bad, just a number), they attach to it their beliefs or myths about or perceptions of how good or bad they think they look at that given moment on that given day.

It's a never-ending vicious circle that continues to destroy more women's happiness than anyone will ever know.

The woman who looks and truly feels great in her skin listens first and foremost to her body and how she feels. And if she wants some external feedback, she'll use two powerful things: the mirror and her clothes.

Much like the scale, the mirror simply shows how her body looks at that given hour, at that given moment, on that given day.

Just a few hours later, she can look different. Yet, she also knows that her judgment of what she sees colors how she thinks her body looks.

She's wise enough to know that the image she sees after having a tough day at work could very well be different from the one she sees after just receiving some great news.

She also understands that not every mirror reflects the same kind of image. Some mirrors distort the body by making it look bigger, while others make it look smaller. She's wise enough to know that the mirror can be trusted, but only to a certain point.

The other method for judging her weight—the one that we prefer she use—is her clothes, especially old pants, skirts, or belts.

And while clothes (especially denim) can shrink when first washed and fit much tighter the first time they're worn, she'll try on that old belt or clothes if she ever wonders about her body size (not her body image).

If those clothes don't fit like she'd like them to, she can decide whether losing weight or firming up is important or not at that time in her life. If she decides it is important, she can adjust her thinking, diet, and exercise to ensure that her body will fit into them more easily in the future.

As always, it's she, not her body, who's in total control of her life and how she feels about it.

That's just the way it should be.

Tip #14 Take-Away:
Keep the old clothes, but toss the scale.

SWEET 16 TIP #15—KNOW WHY YOU HAVE A BODY

Women, more so than men, are said to have an amazing ability to be intuitive. Women's intuition, they call it. And this is the case when it comes to their bodies and knowing why they have them. Yes, women are life givers; our mothers gave birth to all of us.

But women with healthy minds and bodies take the whole intuition thing a big leap further when they truly understand and appreciate why they were given the genes they were given and the bodies they have or have the potential to have if they desire.

Certainly, many women care about their looks, but the ones with the healthiest minds and bodies put their outward appearance in the right perspective.

They don't so much care what their bodies look like cosmetically as they do that their bodies work the way they want them to so they can freely and easily do whatever they need to do.

This is a significant difference between women who are obsessed with their looks and body and those who are in control of them.

Those in control of their bodies know that they not only carry around their brains and do everything their brains tell them to do or not do, they also are their mode of transportation—their earthly cars, so to speak—that takes them from point A to point B and anywhere else they wish to go.

Whenever it gets harder to use their bodies to do the activities and things they like to do, women with healthy bodies and minds will either eat less or do more activity or, for faster results, a little of both at the same time until they get their bodies back to the way they want them to feel.

The body is meant to serve you. You are not a servant to it.

Learn a lesson from the women who look and feel great: Keep your thinking about your body and why you have it in the right perspective and balance and it will be your faithful servant for the rest of your life.

Tip #15 Take-Away:
The body you have is yours for life, so treat it well.

SWEET 16 TIP #16—GRADUALLY COMBINE ALL THE TIPS FOR SPECTACULAR RESULTS

Women who look and feel great don't do just one or two things.

They do many little things, and when you put those little things together, you come up with very powerful ingredients that make up a very powerful recipe we call the Sweet 16 formula for success.

If you've ever made a cake, you know that it doesn't matter if you live in India or Indiana, London or New York, or Paris, France, or Paris, Texas—if you use the same ingredients and follow the same directions, you'll always get the same results.

And it's the same for the Sweet 16 formula for success.

In addition to the 15 tips you've read about, we'd like you to also do this:

- Leave the table a little hungry—never full.

- Make only little adjustments to your exercise and diet at any one time so you can better determine what works and what doesn't.

- Add the 15 ingredients you just discovered to your life and start using them today to make a big difference in how your body looks and feels tomorrow.

As we told you, if you want good results, try using a few of the ingredients at first. Then, add another ingredient for slightly better results.

Keep adding those ingredients—slowly at first, there's no hurry since you'll have the rest of your life to enjoy them—until you're easily using all of the ingredients in the Sweet 16. *Remember: a few ingredients for good results, more ingredients for better results.*

And we want you to do something different this time. Don't expect much. Rather, get your mind off of whether it will work or not or how quickly or well it will work for you. You've done that in the past and look how it's made you feel.

Rarely does reality exceed our expectations. However, not expecting too much and simply doing the things the Sweet 16 say to do will create the calm environment your brain (the unconscious) needs and works best in, resulting in the changes you want deep down inside.

Trust in this.

Think about it: In your past, when there was something you really wanted to happen and you thought about it for a very long time, did it ever come? The old saying "A watched pot never boils" is so true.

But what happened when you told yourself, "Forget it. I'm not going to worry myself or think about it anymore." Didn't it seem like the results you wanted came to you quickly and in ways you may not have expected?

The women who we told you about in the Sweet 16 told us that's one of the reasons they've been so successful at losing the weight or keeping themselves at the same weight—some for more than 60 years.

Tip #16 Take-Away:
Get out of your own way and let the Sweet 16 tips work
their magic.

Our best wishes for the great body and wonderful life that await you!

How to Read a Food Label Like a Pro

The FDA is at the vanguard in helping Americans make healthy choices about food and diet. This information is available on the FDA's Web site, but for your ease of reference, I'm including it in this Bonus Section. Straight from the source!

HOW TO UNDERSTAND AND USE THE NUTRITION FACTS LABEL

People look at food labels for different reasons. But whatever the reason, many consumers would like to know how to use this information more effectively and easily. The following label-building skills are intended to make it easier for you to use nutrition labels to make quick, informed food choices that contribute to a healthy diet.

THE NUTRITION FACTS LABEL—AN OVERVIEW

The information in the main or top section (see #1–4 and #6 on the sample nutrition label on page 166) can vary with each food product;

Source: *The following 12 pages are courtesy of US Food and Drug Administration, November 2004.*

it contains product-specific information (serving size, calories, and nutrient information). The bottom part (see #5 on the sample label below) contains a footnote with Daily Values (DVs) for 2,000- and 2,500-calorie diets. This footnote provides recommended dietary information for important nutrients, including fats, sodium, and fiber. The footnote is found only on larger packages and does not change from product to product.

In the following Nutrition Facts label we have shaded certain sections to help you focus on those areas that will be explained in detail. You will not see these shadings on the food labels on products you purchase.

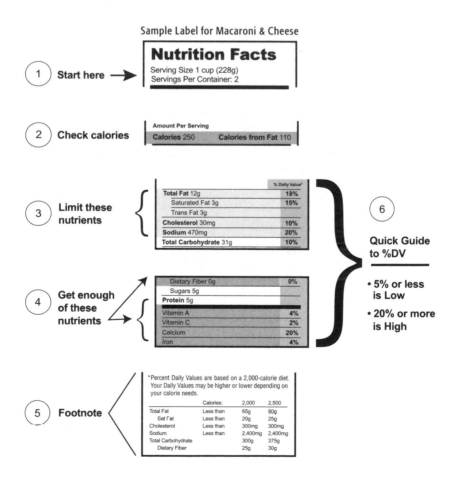

Sample Label for Macaroni & Cheese

① The Serving Size

| Serving Size 1 cup (228g) |
| Servings Per Container: 2 |

The first place to start when you look at the Nutrition Facts label is the serving size and the number of servings in the package. Serving sizes are standardized to make it easier to compare similar foods; they are provided in familiar units, such as cups or pieces, followed by the metric amount, e.g., the number of grams.

The size of the serving on the food package influences the number of calories and all the nutrient amounts listed on the top part of the label. **Pay attention to the serving size, especially how many servings there are in the food package. Then ask yourself, "How many servings am I consuming?" (e.g., ½ serving, 1 serving, or more).** In the sample label, one serving of macaroni and cheese equals 1 cup. If you ate the whole package, you would eat **2** cups. That doubles the calories and other nutrient numbers, including the Percent Daily Values (%DV) as shown in the example on this page.

Example				
	Single Serving	%DV	Double Serving	%DV
Serving Size	1 cup (228g)		2 cups (456g)	
Calories	250		500	
Calories from Fat	110		220	
Total Fat	12g	18%	24g	36%
Trans Fat	1.5g		3g	
Saturated Fat	3g	15%	6g	30%
Cholesterol	30mg	10%	60mg	20%
Sodium	470mg	20%	940mg	40%
Total Carbohydrate	31g	10%	62g	20%
Dietary Fiber	0g	0%	0g	0%
Sugars	5g		10g	
Protein	5g		10g	
Vitamin A		4%		8%
Vitamin C		2%		4%
Calcium		20%		40%
Iron		4%		8%

② Calories (and Calories from Fat)

Calories provide a measure of how much energy you get from a serving of this food. Many Americans consume more calories than they need without meeting recommended intakes for a number of nutrients.

The calorie section of the label can help you manage your weight (i.e., gain, lose, or maintain). **Remember: the number of servings you consume determines the number of calories you actually eat (your portion amount).**

Amount Per Serving	
Calories 250	**Calories from Fat** 110

In the example, there are 250 calories in one serving of this macaroni and cheese. How many calories from fat are there in ONE serving? Answer: 110 calories, which means almost half the calories in a single serving come from fat. What if you ate the whole package content? Then, you would consume two servings, or 500 calories, and 220 would come from fat.

GENERAL GUIDE TO CALORIES

- 40 calories is low

- 100 calories is moderate

- 400 calories or more is high

The **General Guide to Calories** provides a general reference for calories when you look at a Nutrition Facts label. This guide is based on a 2,000-calorie diet.

③ ④ THE NUTRIENTS: HOW MUCH?

Look at the top of the nutrient section in the sample label. It shows you some key nutrients that impact on your health and separates them into two main groups:

LIMIT THESE NUTRIENTS

Total Fat 12g		18%
Saturated Fat 3g		15%
Trans Fat 3g		
Cholesterol 30mg		10%
Sodium 470mg		20%

The nutrients that are listed first are the ones Americans generally eat in adequate amounts, or even too much. They are identified as **Limit These**

Nutrients. Eating too much fat, saturated fat, trans fat, cholesterol, or sodium may increase your risk of certain chronic diseases, like heart disease, some cancers, or high blood pressure.

Important: Health experts recommend that you keep your intake of saturated fat, trans fat, and cholesterol as low as possible as part of a nutritionally balanced diet.

GET ENOUGH OF THESE NUTRIENTS

Dietary Fiber 0g	0%
Vitamin A	4%
Vitamin C	2%
Calcium	20%
Iron	4%

Most Americans don't get enough dietary fiber, vitamin A, vitamin C, calcium, and iron in their diets. They are identified as **Get Enough of These Nutrients.** Eating enough of these nutrients can improve your health and help reduce the risk of some diseases and conditions. For example, getting enough calcium may reduce the risk of osteoporosis, a condition that results in brittle bones as one ages (see calcium section on page 174). Eating a diet high in dietary fiber promotes healthy bowel function. Additionally, a diet rich in fruits, vegetables, and grain products that contain dietary fiber, particularly soluble fiber, and low in saturated fat and cholesterol may reduce the risk of heart disease.

Remember: You can use the Nutrition Facts label not only to help limit those nutrients you want to cut back on but also to increase those nutrients you need to consume in greater amounts.

⑤ UNDERSTANDING THE FOOTNOTE ON THE BOTTOM OF THE NUTRITION FACTS LABEL

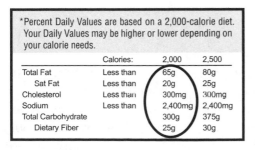

Note the asterisk used after the heading "% Daily Value" on the Nutrition Facts label. It refers to the **Footnote** in the lower part of the nutrition label, which tells you **"%DVs are based on a 2,000-calorie diet."**

This statement must be on all food labels. But the remaining information in the full footnote may not be on the package if the size of the label is too small. When the full footnote does appear, it will always be the same. It doesn't change from product to product, because it shows recommended dietary advice for all Americans—it is not about a specific food product.

Look at the amounts circled in the footnote on page 169—these are the Daily Values (DVs) for each nutrient listed and are based on public health experts' advice. DVs are recommended levels of intakes. DVs in the footnote are based on a 2,000- or 2,500-calorie diet. Note how the DVs for some nutrients change, while others (for cholesterol and sodium) remain the same for both calorie amounts.

HOW THE DAILY VALUES RELATE TO THE %DVS

Look at the example below for another way to see how the DVs relate to the %DVs and dietary guidance. For each nutrient listed there is a DV, a %DV, and dietary advice or a goal. If you follow this dietary advice, you will stay within public health experts' recommended upper or lower limits for the nutrients listed, based on a 2,000-calorie daily diet.

Examples of DVs versus %DVs
Based on a 2,000-Calorie Diet

NUTRIENT	DV	%DV	GOAL
Total Fat	65g	= 100%DV	Less than
Sat Fat	20g	= 100%DV	Less than
Cholesterol	300mg	= 100%DV	Less than
Sodium	2,400mg	= 100%DV	Less than
Total Carbohydrate	300g	= 100%DV	At least
Dietary Fiber	25g	= 100%DV	At least

Upper Limit—Eat "Less Than" . . .

The nutrients that have "upper daily limits" are listed first on the footnote of larger labels and on the example above. Upper limits means it is recommended that you stay below—eat "less than"—the Daily Value nutrient amounts listed per day. For example, the DV for saturated fat is 20g. This amount is 100%DV for this nutrient. So what is the goal or dietary advice? To eat "less than" 20g or 100%DV for the day.

Lower Limit—Eat "At Least" . . .

Now look at the section where dietary fiber is listed. The DV for dietary fiber is 25g, which is 100%DV. This means it is recommended that you eat "at least" this amount of dietary fiber per day.

The DV for total carbohydrate is 300g or 100%DV. This amount is recommended for a balanced daily diet that is based on 2,000 calories, but can vary, depending on your daily intake of fat and protein.

Now let's look at the %DVs.

⑥ The Percent Daily Value (%DV)

% Daily Value*
18%
15%
10%
20%
10%
0%
4%
2%
20%
4%

The % Daily Values (%DVs) are based on the Daily Value recommendations for key nutrients but only for a 2,000-calorie daily diet—not 2,500 calories. You, like most people, may not know how many calories you consume in a day. But you can still use the %DV as a frame of reference whether or not you consume more or less than 2,000 calories.

The %DV helps you determine if a serving of food is high or low in a nutrient. Note: a few nutrients, like trans fat, do not have a %DV— they will be discussed later.

Do you need to know how to calculate percentages to use the %DV? No, the label (the %DV) does the math for you. It helps you interpret the numbers (grams and milligrams) by putting them all on the same scale for the day (0–100%DV). The %DV column doesn't add up vertically to 100%. Instead each nutrient is based on 100% of the daily requirements for that nutrient (for a 2,000-calorie diet). This way you can tell high from low and know which nutrients contribute a lot, or a little, to your **daily** recommended allowance (upper or lower).

QUICK GUIDE TO THE %DV

5%DV or less is low and 20%DV or more is high.

	% Daily Value*
Total Fat 12g	**18%**
Saturated Fat 3g	**15%**
Trans Fat 3g	
Cholesterol 30mg	**10%**
Sodium 470mg	**20%**
Total Carbohydrate 31g	**10%**
Dietary Fiber 0g	**0%**
Sugars 5g	
Protein 5g	
Vitamin A	**4%**
Vitamin C	**2%**
Calcium	**20%**
Iron	**4%**

This guide tells you that **5%DV or less is low** for all nutrients, those you want to limit (e.g., fat, saturated fat, cholesterol, and sodium), or for those that you want to consume in greater amounts (fiber, calcium, etc.). As the **Quick Guide** shows, **20%DV or more is high** for all nutrients.

> *Example:* Look at the amount of Total Fat in one serving listed on the sample nutrition label. Is 18%DV contributing a lot or a little to your fat limit of 100%DV? Check the **Quick Guide to %DV.** 18%DV, which is below 20%DV, is not yet high, but what if you ate the whole package (two servings)? You would double that amount, eating 36% of your daily allowance for Total Fat. Coming from just one food, that amount leaves you with 64% of your fat allowance (100% – 36% = 64%) for *all* of the other foods you eat that day, snacks and drinks included.

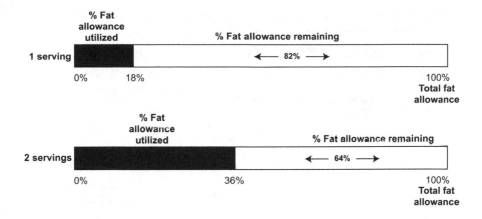

USING THE %DV

COMPARISONS: The %DV also makes it easy for you to make comparisons. You can compare one product or brand to a similar product. Just make sure the serving sizes are similar, especially the weight (e.g., grams, milligrams, ounces) of each product. It's easy to see which foods are higher or lower in nutrients because the serving sizes are generally consistent for similar types of foods (see the comparison example on page 177), except in a few cases like cereals.

NUTRIENT CONTENT CLAIMS: Use the %DV to help you quickly distinguish one claim from another, such as "reduced fat" versus "light" or "nonfat." Just compare the %DVs for Total Fat in each food product to see which one is higher or lower in that nutrient—**there is no need to memorize definitions.** This works when comparing all nutrient content claims, such as "less," "light," "low," "free," "more," "high," etc.

DIETARY TRADE-OFFS: You can **use the %DV to help you make dietary trade-offs** with other foods throughout the day. You don't have to give up a favorite food to eat a healthy diet. When a food you like is high in fat, balance it with foods that are low in fat at other times of the day. Also, pay attention to how much you eat so that the **total** amount of fat for the day stays below 100%DV.

NUTRIENTS WITH A %DV BUT NO WEIGHT LISTED: CALCIUM

Nutrition Facts

Serving Size 1 cup (236ml)
Servings Per Container: 1

Amount Per Serving

Calories 80   **Calories from Fat** 0

                                    % Daily Value*

Total Fat 0g	0%
Saturated Fat 0g	0%
Trans Fat 0g	
Cholesterol Less than 5mg	0%
Sodium 120mg	0%
Total Carbohydrate 11g	4%
Dietary Fiber 0g	0%
Sugars 11g	
Protein 9g	17%

Vitamin A 10%   •   Vitamin C 4%
Calcium 30%   •   Iron 0%   •   Vitamin D 25%

*Percent Daily Values are based on a 2,000-calorie diet.
Your Daily Values may be higher or lower depending on
your calorie needs.

CALCIUM: Look at the %DV for calcium on food packages so you know how much one serving contributes to the *total amount you need* per day. Remember, a food with 20%DV or more contributes a lot of calcium to your daily total, while one with 5%DV or less contributes a little.

Experts advise adult consumers to consume adequate amounts of calcium, that is, 1,000mg or 100%DV in a daily 2,000-calorie diet. This advice is often given in milligrams (mg), but the Nutrition Facts label **only** lists a %DV for calcium.

For certain populations, they advise that adolescents, especially girls, consume 1,300mg (130%DV) and post-menopausal women consume 1,200mg (120%DV) of calcium daily. The DV for calcium on food labels is 1,000mg.

Don't be fooled. Always check the label for calcium because you can't make assumptions about the amount of calcium in specific food categories. Example: the amount of calcium in milk, whether skim or whole, is generally the same per serving, whereas the amount of calcium in the same size yogurt container (8 oz) can vary from 20–45%DV.

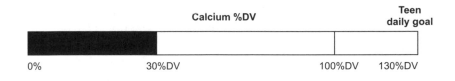

	Calcium %DV		Teen daily goal

0%   30%DV   100%DV   130%DV

Equivalencies

30% DV = 300mg calcium = 1 cup of milk

100% DV = 1,000mg calcium

130% DV = 1,300mg calcium

NUTRIENTS WITHOUT A %DV: TRANS FATS, PROTEIN, AND SUGARS

Note that trans fat, sugars, and protein do not list a %DV on the Nutrition Facts label.

Plain Yogurt   Fruit Yogurt

Nutrition Facts	
Serving Size 1 Container (226g)	
Servings Per Container: 1	
Amount Per Serving	
Calories 110	**Calories from Fat** 0
	% Daily Value*
Total Fat 0g	0%
Saturated Fat 0g	0%
Trans Fat 0g	
Cholesterol Less than 5mg	1%
Sodium 160mg	7%
Total Carbohydrate 15g	5%
Dietary Fiber 0g	0%
Sugars 10g	
Protein 13g	
Vitamin A 0% • Vitamin C 4%	
Calcium 45% • Iron 0%	
*Percent Daily Values are based on a 2,000-calorie diet. Your Daily Values may be higher or lower depending on your calorie needs.	

Nutrition Facts	
Serving Size 1 Container (227g)	
Servings Per Container: 1	
Amount Per Serving	
Calories 240	**Calories from Fat** 25
	% Daily Value*
Total Fat 3g	4%
Saturated Fat 1.5g	9%
Trans Fat 0g	
Cholesterol 15mg	5%
Sodium 140mg	6%
Total Carbohydrate 46g	15%
Dietary Fiber Less than 1g	3%
Sugars 44g	
Protein 9g	
Vitamin A 2% • Vitamin C 4%	
Calcium 35% • Iron 0%	
*Percent Daily Values are based on a 2,000-calorie diet. Your Daily Values may be higher or lower depending on your calorie needs.	

TRANS FAT: Experts could not provide a reference value for trans fat nor any other information that FDA believes is sufficient to establish a Daily Value or %DV. Scientific reports link trans fat (and saturated fat) with raising blood LDL ("bad") cholesterol levels, both of which increase your risk of coronary heart disease, a leading cause of death in the US.

Important: Health experts recommend that you keep your intake of saturated fat, trans fat, and cholesterol as low as possible as part of a nutritionally balanced diet.

PROTEIN: A %DV is required to be listed if a claim is made for protein, such as "high in protein." Otherwise, unless the food is meant for use by infants and children under 4 years old, none is needed. Current scientific evidence indicates that protein intake is not a public health concern for adults and children over 4 years of age.

SUGARS: No daily reference value has been established for sugars because no recommendations have been made for the total amount to eat in a day. Keep in mind that the sugars listed on the Nutrition Facts label include naturally occurring sugars (like those in fruit and milk) as well as those added to a food or drink. Check the ingredient list for specifics on added sugars.

Take a look at the nutrients section of the Nutrition Fact labels for the two yogurt examples. The plain yogurt on the left has 10g of sugars, while the fruit yogurt on the right has 44g of sugars in one serving.

Now look below at the ingredient lists for the two yogurts. Ingredients are listed in descending order of weight (from most to least). Note that no added sugars or sweeteners are in the list of ingredients for the plain yogurt, yet 10g of sugars were listed on the Nutrition Facts label. This is because there are no added sugars in plain yogurt, only naturally occurring sugars (lactose in the milk).

Plain Yogurt—Contains No Added Sugars

INGREDIENTS: CULTURED PASTEURIZED GRADE A NONFAT MILK, WHEY PROTEIN CONCENTRATE, PECTIN, CARAGEENAN.

Fruit Yogurt—Contains Added Sugars

INGREDIENTS: CULTURED GRADE A REDUCED FAT MILK, APPLES, HIGH FRUCTOSE CORN SYRUP, CINNAMON, NUTMEG, NATURAL FLAVORS, AND PECTIN. CONTAINS ACTIVE YOGURT AND L. ACIDOPHILUS CULTURES

If you are concerned about your intake of sugars, make sure that added sugars are not listed as one of the first few ingredients. Other names for added sugars include: corn syrup, high-fructose corn syrup, fruit juice concentrate, maltose, dextrose, sucrose, honey, and maple syrup.

To limit nutrients that have no %DV, like trans fat and sugars, compare the labels of similar products and choose the food with the lowest amount.

COMPARISON EXAMPLE

Below are two kinds of milk. One is reduced fat milk, and the other is nonfat milk. Each serving size is 1 cup. Which has more calories and more saturated fat? Which one has more calcium?

Reduced Fat Milk
2% Milkfat

Nonfat Milk

Nutrition Facts

Serving Size 1 cup (236ml)
Servings Per Container: 1

Amount Per Serving

Calories 120	Calories from Fat 45

	% Daily Value*
Total Fat 5g	8%
Saturated Fat 3g	15%
Trans Fat 0g	
Cholesterol 20mg	7%
Sodium 120mg	5%
Total Carbohydrate 11g	4%
Dietary Fiber 0g	0%
Sugars 11g	
Protein 9g	17%

Vitamin A 10%	•	Vitamin C 4%
Calcium 30%	•	Vitamin D 25%

*Percent Daily Values are based on a 2,000-calorie diet. Your Daily Values may be higher or lower depending on your calorie needs.

Nutrition Facts

Serving Size 1 cup (236ml)
Servings Per Container: 1

Amount Per Serving

Calories 80	Calories from Fat 0

	% Daily Value*
Total Fat 0g	0%
Saturated Fat 0g	0%
Trans Fat 0g	
Cholesterol Less than 5mg	0%
Sodium 120mg	5%
Total Carbohydrate 11g	4%
Dietary Fiber 0g	0%
Sugars 11g	
Protein 9g	17%

Vitamin A 10%	•	Vitamin C 4%
Calcium 30%	• Iron 0% •	Vitamin D 25%

*Percent Daily Values are based on a 2,000-calorie diet. Your Daily Values may be higher or lower depending on your calorie needs.

Answer: As you can see, they both have the same amount of calcium, but the nonfat milk has no saturated fat and has 40 calories less per serving than the reduced fat milk.

In addition to all of these great resources from the FDA, here are a few bonus tips straight from the authors of *Menopause Reset!*

Food Marketing Deceptions

Let me tell you about some common food marketing practices that on the surface may look harmless, but can be big no-nos for helping you lose weight and keep it off.

Whole Milk versus 2% Milk

How many people do you know who won't drink regular milk because they think it's fattening, yet they'll drink gallons of 2% milk?

Time for a little surprise.

First, the numbers.

In 1 cup of whole milk there are 150 calories, and in 2% milk there are 120 calories.

There are 8 fat grams in whole milk. In 2% milk there are 5 fat grams.

Whole milk contains 72 fat calories, while 2% milk contains 45 fat calories.

That means whole milk gets 48 percent of its calories from fat.

So, with 2% milk being merely 2 percent fat, it's the better choice to drink, right?

Surprise!

Two percent milk gets 37.5 percent of its calories from fat!

And look at how long we've been drinking it, thinking all the while that we're keeping our fat intake low.

The truth is, the only difference between whole milk and 2% milk is 3 grams of fat per glass.

When it comes to whole milk or 2%, it's your decision whether you want to use 8 grams or 5 grams of the 30 grams of fat you're allowed per day.

But, that's only one factor to consider.

The cholesterol level differs greatly between whole and 2% milk, with 33 milligrams found in whole milk and 18 milligrams in 2% milk.

Here are the numbers:

	1 Cup Whole Milk	1 Cup 2% Milk
Calories	150	120
Fat grams	8	5
Calories from fat	48%	37.5%

BUTTER VERSUS MARGARINE

One of the most-asked questions for nutritionists is: Which is better, butter or margarine?

The answer, as far as fat content is concerned, will surprise you.

The *only* difference between butter and margarine is the amount of *cholesterol* they contain.

I believe that to most of us, butter is tastier. And if you do not have a cholesterol problem, I do not see a reason to avoid butter. Remember, moderation is the answer, and not deprivation.

Whenever you use butter, be aware of how many grams of fat are in the amount you are using, and calculate it into your 30 grams of fat per day allowance.

Here are the numbers:

	1 Tbsp. Butter	1 Tbsp. Margarine
Calories	100	100
Fat grams	11	11
Calories from fat	99%	99%
Cholesterol	31 mg	0 mg

Now take a look at the differences between margarine and spreads such as I Can't Believe It's Not Butter!

	1 Tbsp. Margarine	1 Tbsp. Spread
Calories	100	50
Fat grams	11	5
Calories from fat	99%	90%

The end result is that, yes, you'll be ingesting 6 fewer grams of fat if you choose 1 tablespoon of spread, but the fat content is still 90 percent of the total calories!

Again, don't look at the calories. Look at the *amount of grams of fat* you're giving your body and make sure that it does not go higher than 30 grams of fat per day.

OIL VERSUS OIL: VEGETABLE, CORN, OR OLIVE?

Oil is oil is oil! Labeling descriptors such as "no cholesterol," "all natural," and "light" are grossly misleading if you're looking to determine the nutritional value of these products. Any oil product gives your body a 100 percent shot of fat. Remember that, and use it in moderation.

If you do use oil, choose the one that is the highest in monounsaturated fats, such as olive oil. The rate of heart attacks in the Mediterranean region, where olive oil is a staple, is lower than elsewhere in the Western world. The rates of breast and colon cancer are lower in Spain and Greece, where olive oil is king. Therefore, if you do use oil in moderation, for better taste and health choose olive oil.

SNEAKY CEREAL SECRETS

When it comes to cereal, mysteries abound. The first question is: Where's the fruit? Many cereal boxes show heaping bowlfuls of fruit, yet it often turns out that there is little fruit inside the box. Kellogg's Fruitful Bran, for example, contains 1.3 ounces of fruit, which is less than 1 cup.

I suggest adding your own fruit instead and not paying extra for cereal that claims to have it.

WHAT DID YOU SAY, HONEY?

Honey tastes great, and because it has such a healthful image, cereal makers use it extensively in product names like General Mills's Honey Nut Cheerios, Kellogg's Honey Smacks, Kellogg's Nut and Honey Crunch, and the list goes on.

The truth is that the body processes honey like it does sugar, so just be smart and don't go overboard using honey to make anything and everything sweet.

FIBER AND CRUNCH

Here is another marketing ploy that food makers use a lot. The first thing you need to know is that you can't assume that a cereal is high in fiber just because the name sounds fibrous. Nut and Honey Crunch, General Mills's Crispy Wheats 'n Raisins, Kellogg's Rice Krispies, and Post's Golden Crisp are low in fiber.

And what about the sugar?

Although their names might have been changed, the sugar levels in several breakfast cereals have not been reduced. Kellogg's Sugar Pops is now Corn Pops, and Kellogg's Sugar Smacks is now Honey Smacks. But they're still high in sugar.

IT'S ALL ABOUT BEING A SMART LABEL READER

There is no doubt that advertising and labeling information can help you make wise and healthy food selections if you know what to look for.

How many times have you seen or heard ads for brands of vegetable oil that say they are "low cholesterol"? It's no surprise that when most people see that, they think that the other brands of vegetable oil have cholesterol, yet the truth is, no vegetable oil does. Cholesterol is found only in foods from animals.

And then there are the little-known oils that so many food companies use in their products that can really wreak havoc on a body. These oils are the real biggies when it comes to contributing the most saturated fats to Western-style diets, and they are coconut oil and palm kernel oil—both vegetable fats. Most women don't realize that these two oils can raise cholesterol levels and clog coronary arteries faster than animal fats.

Nutrition and Exercise Myths and Truths

For any woman, especially the menopausal woman, the daily barrage of nutrition, exercise, and latest research news can be overwhelming. There's so much information and from so many sources. What's true and what's not?

Then there's those pesky things called myths that keep getting repeated year after year and, seemingly, without anyone questioning if what they're hearing and reading is true.

Relax.

I've done the work for you.

Here are seven of the biggest myths I've heard my patients repeating and the answers I tell them that keep them on the road to excellent results.

The first . . .

MYTH #1: SHELLFISH HAS TOO MUCH CHOLESTEROL

I couldn't even begin to tell you how many times women have told me that shellfish (such as shrimp, lobster, and so forth) are loaded with cholesterol and, therefore, harmful to their health. And where

183

do you think these wonderful women patients of mine heard such pronouncements? Try from their physicians and cardiologists.

So is it true?

The Truth: Not true.

To begin with, shellfish contains high levels of protein and low levels of fats, thereby making it a very healthy food choice.

In addition, three large prawns (shrimp) will have only 180 to 200 milligrams (mg) of cholesterol.

Compare that to the 140 mg of cholesterol found in one small chicken breast or the 180 mg of cholesterol in one chicken thigh.

Keep in mind that 70 to 80 percent of your total cholesterol number comes from cholesterol produced by your own liver, and only 20 to 30 percent of your body's cholesterol is influenced by your food intake.

Bottom Line: Enjoy your shellfish with lemon and skip the butter.

MYTH #2: WALKING DOESN'T HELP SPEED WEIGHT LOSS

During my more than 20 years in practice, I have had many women tell me emphatically that just walking isn't enough exercise to help them lose weight.

With so many of them saying and believing it, it must be correct, right?

The Truth: How wrong they are!

Thousands of times, my patients keep proving over and over that simply walking, and only walking, is highly effective at helping them lose weight and keep the weight off.

Bottom Line: Our bodies were made to walk. And best of all, you don't need to buy expensive equipment or join a gym to do it. All you need is a good pair of walking shoes and a daily walk of at least 30 minutes each day, and you will be on the road to great results.

MYTH #3: YOU MUST USE DIFFERENT EXERCISES AND EQUIPMENT TO GET GOOD RESULTS

On the surface, this statement appears to have some truth to it. For many people, they get bored very quickly doing the same workout over and over, and it's no wonder that they lose motivation and stop. So, for those people whose bodies habituate quickly (get accustomed to any new exercise or workout) and they want to change what they do when they work out, I say go for it!

But do you need to do that to burn more calories?

The Truth: A workout session that burns 350 calories is the same workout output if it is done on the treadmill, the elliptical, or walking or jogging in the street. If the body burns a total of 350 calories for a given workout session, that 350 calories is the same number of calories that will be achieved regardless of what mode of exercise or combination of them is used to do it.

Bottom Line: Keep in mind that different types of exercises and workouts can burn those 350 faster or slower, but if the goal is simply to burn 350 calories in a workout, the thermogenic effect of exercise (TEE) is the same no matter what exercise machine is used.

MYTH #4: DIFFERENT KINDS OF FRUITS AND VEGETABLES HAVE TOO MANY SUGARS, SO YOU SHOULD AVOID THEM

Many times I've heard people tell me, "Don't eat baby carrots because there is too much sugar in them" or "Don't eat grapes (or melons or bananas) because all the sugar in it will make you gain weight."

Well, it is true that fruits and vegetables have sugars, so are they right?

The Truth: Yes, fruits and veggies do have sugars, but they are natural sugars and not processed sugars, and that makes a huge difference.

Eating natural sugars (e.g., fruits and veggies in 100- to 120-calorie servings) helps regulate blood sugar and helps prevent insulin production and secretion into the blood. All of which helps the body burn fat more efficiently.

Compare that to what processed sugars do: They trigger increases in blood sugar levels, insulin production, and fat storage. Most women don't gain weight from just eating berries. Put a little fresh cream on them, and it can change everything.

Bottom Line: Eating more fruits and veggies throughout the day (within reason and not more total calories than your body needs each day) can help you have more energy and help better regulate your body's blood sugar level, which can help keep you in the fat-burning and weight loss zone.

MYTH #5: TO LOSE FAT, YOU MUST SWEAT WHEN YOU EXERCISE

The myth says it all.

But is it true?

The Truth: Yes, finishing a hard, sweaty exercise session can make you feel great, powerful, and unstoppable, but do you need to do it in order to give your body the most-efficient fat-burning workout?

No.

It boils down to workout intensity and which energy sources the body best uses to achieve the workout goal: fat burning.

During a workout, the body utilizes three major energy sources for the muscles to contract: fats, glucose (sugars in the blood), and glycogen (sugars in the liver and in the muscles).

At the beginning of any exercise routine (during the first 12 to 18 minutes), the body utilizes more sugars than fat. After that time period, the body will shift its energy usage to more fats than sugars. However, the intensity of the cardiovascular workout will also determine how much fat will be burned.

A workout intensity of 50 to 70 percent of maximum capacity or target heart rate (THR) is the most efficient for fat burning. A higher intensity level of 70 to 85 percent provides an excellent workout for cardiovascular conditioning and benefits, but it is not as efficient for fat burning.

Bottom Line: You don't need to work out hard to burn fat.

MYTH #6: STAY AWAY FROM BAGELS BECAUSE THEY HAVE TOO MANY CARBS

That myth is only the beginning.

"Bagels have too many carbs and you can't lose weight if you eat them" and "Bagels have too many calories and lots of sugar" are two others that women keep on believing.

Good thing no one has told my patients, because they are still eating bagels. So am I missing something here?

The Truth: If you ask my patients, they'll emphatically tell you "no!" because they are still enjoying their daily bagel and losing weight and keeping it off.

Let's take a look at the bagel.

It has carbs, some vegetarian protein, fiber, and very little fat. So far so good. Depending on the bagel size, an average bagel has about 300 calories, 1 to 2 grams of fat, 6 to 7 grams of protein, and the rest of it is carbohydrates.

So, you might be asking that if you are eating a half of a bagel with a little all-fruit jam on it, what's wrong with having those 200 calories?

I say nothing!

Compare that to a typical breakfast that is a bowl of cereal (150 to 250 calories from mostly carbs), with 3 to 4 ounces of milk (calories depending on type of milk), and you would be consuming the same amount of calories that are found in one bagel.

And if you are eating a bacon and cheese egg sandwich, or bacon and cheese omelet, a bagel can be just half of the calories of what's contained in those breakfasts.

Bottom Line: Go ahead and have your bagel. Just don't load it with cream cheese or butter.

MYTH #7: STRENGTH TRAINING IS ALL YOU NEED TO BURN FAT

This is a common statement I hear people repeat. Two closely related others are "The more muscle you have, the more you'll burn fat" and "Stop doing cardiovascular training and just increase your strength exercise program, and that's all you'll need to burn fat."

They sound believable, but just how much so?

The Truth: The increase of lean body mass is one of the physiological mechanisms that help increase metabolism and daily metabolic rate (DMR), and positively affect caloric output and weight loss.

An increase in muscle tone and size will positively affect bone density. A denser bone and a toner muscle will increase caloric output every second, minute, and hour of the day, all of which helps elevate DMR and enhance weight loss.

A good thing, right?

Well, unless you're a celebrity or a bodybuilder who makes the gym their second home, just basing your exercise program on doing something that will increase your lean body mass can take a long time, especially getting your lean body mass to the point where it begins to significantly affect metabolism and weight loss.

Most women I know simply don't have the time or desire to do that.

However, the good news is that you don't need to live in the gym or exercise for hours to make positive changes to your body's lean body mass and help prevent osteoporosis.

Bottom Line: If you're already not doing so, begin adding strength training to your weekly workouts, but do so in addition to your cardiovascular training. For best results, you should do them both.

Selected Literature, Research, and References

Abete, I., D. Parra, and J. A. Martinez. "Energy-Restricted Diets Based on a Distinct Food Selection Affecting the Glycemic Index Induce Different Weight Loss and Oxidative Response." *Clin Nutr* 2008;27(4):545–51.

Astrup, A., T. M. Larsen, and A. Harper. "Atkins and Other Low-Carbohydrate Diets: Hoax or an Effective Tool for Weight Loss?" *Lancet* 2004;364(9437):897–99.

Astrup, A., S. Madsbad, L. Breum, T. J. Jensen, J. P. Kroustrup, and T. M. Larsen. "Effect of Tesofensine on Bodyweight Loss, Body Composition, and Quality of Life in Obese Patients: A Randomised, Double-Blind, Placebo-Controlled Trial." *Lancet* 2008;372(9653):1906–13.

Astrup, A., S. S. Toubro, A. Raben, and A. R. Skov. "The Role of Low-Fat Diets and Fat Substitutes in Body Weight Management: What Have We Learned from Clinical Studies?" *J Am Diet Assoc* 1997;97(7):S82–87.

Bazarra-Fernández, A. "Postmenopausal Osteoporosis and Weight Gain." *Bone* 2008;43(Suppl 1):S124.

Bergouignan, A., and S. Blanc. "The Energetics of Obesity." *J Soc Biol* 2006;200(1):29–35.

Blaak, E. E., M. A. van Baak, A. D. M. Kester, and W. H. M. Saris. "ß-adrenergically Mediated Thermogenic and Heart Rate Responses: Effect of Obesity and Weight Loss." *Metabolism* 1995;44(4):520–24.

Brownell, K. D., and J. Rodin. "Medical, Metabolic, and Psychological Effects of Weight Cycling." *Arch Intern Med* 1994;154(12):1325–30.

Casas-Agustench, P., P. López-Uriarte, M. Bulló, E. Ros, A. Gómez-Flores, and J. Salas-Salvadó. "Acute Effects of Three High-Fat Meals with Different Fat Saturations on Energy Expenditure, Substrate Oxidation and Satiety." *Clin Nutr* 2009;28(1):39–45.

Castelo-Branco, C. "Clinical Aspects and Relationships between Weight Gain, Obesity and Menopause." *Maturitas* 2009;63 (Suppl 1):S19.

Claessens, M., W. Calame, A. D. Siemensma, W. H. M. Saris, and M. A. van Baak. "The Thermogenic and Metabolic Effects of Protein Hydrolysate with or without a Carbohydrate Load in Healthy Male Subjects." *Metabolism* 2007;56(8):1051–59.

Colley, R. C., A. P. Hills, N. A. King, and N. M. Byrne. "Exercise-Induced Energy Expenditure: Implications for Exercise Prescription and Obesity." *Patient Educ Couns* 2010;79(3):327–32.

Dubnov, G., A. Brzezinski, and E. M. Berry. "Weight Control and the Management of Obesity after Menopause: The Role of Physical Activity." *Maturitas* 2003;44(2):89–101.

Fogelholm, M., K. Kukkonen-Harjula, A. Nenonen, and M. Pasanen. "Effects of Walking Training on Weight Maintenance after a Very-Low-Energy Diet in Premenopausal Obese Women: A Randomized Controlled Trial." *Arch Intern Med* 2000;160(14): 2177–84.

Gaby, A. R. "Adverse Effects of Dietary Fructose." *Altern Med Rev* 2005;10(4):294–306.

Garry, J. P., and L. M. Whetstone. "Physical Activity and Exercise at Menopause." *Clin Fam Pract* 2002;4(1):53–70.

Grant, S., K. Todd, T. C. Aitchison, P. Kelly, and D. Stoddart. "The Effects of a 12-Week Group Exercise Programme on Physiological and Psychological Variables and Function in Overweight Women." *Public Health* 2004;118(1):31–42.

Gumbiner, B., A. W. Thorburn, and R. R. Henry. "Reduced Glucose-Induced Thermogenesis Is Present in Noninsulin-Dependent Diabetes Mellitus without Obesity." *J Clin Endocrinol Metab* 1995;72(4):801–7.

Hamilton, M. T., D. G. Hamilton, and T. W. Zderic. "Role of Low Energy Expenditure and Sitting in Obesity, Metabolic Syndrome, Type 2 Diabetes, and Cardiovascular Disease." *Diabetes* 2007;56(11):2655–67.

Henriksen, H. B., and S. O. Kolset. "Sugar Intake and Public Health." *Tidsskr Nor Laegeforen* 2007;127(17):2259–62.

Jakicic, J. M., B. H. Marcus, K. I. Gallagher, M. Napolitano, and W. Lang. "Effect of Exercise Duration and Intensity on Weight Loss in Overweight, Sedentary Women: A Randomized Trial." *ACC Curr J Rev* 2004;13(1):21–22.

Jeukendrup, A. E., and S. Aldred. "Fat Supplementation, Health, and Endurance Performance." *Nutrition* 2004;20(7):678–88.

Joubert, L. M., and M. M. Manore. "Exercise, Nutrition, and Homocysteine." *Int J Sport Nutr Exerc Metab* 2006;16(4):341–61.

Judge, B. S., and B. H. Eisenga. "Disorders of Fuel Metabolism: Medical Complications Associated with Starvation, Eating Disorders, Dietary Fads, and Supplements." *Emerg Med Clin North Am* 2005;23(3):789–813.

Kirchengast, S., D. Gruber, M. Sator, and J. Huber. "Postmenopausal Weight Status, Body Composition and Body Fat Distribution in Relation to Parameters of Menstrual and Reproductive History." *Maturitas* 1999;33(2):117–26.

Kohrt, W. M. "Menopause Medicine: Exercise and Weight Gain." *Geriatrics* 2009;64(6):28–29.

Kolasa, K.M. "Weight and Abdominal-Fat Distribution in Menopausal Women." *Clin Fam Pract* 2002;4(1):41–52.

Kong, A., M. L. Neuhouser, L. Xiao, C. M. Ulrich, A. McTiernan, and K. E. Foster-Schubert. "Higher Habitual Intake of Dietary Fat and Carbohydrates Are Associated with Lower Leptin and Higher Ghrelin Concentrations in Overweight and Obese Postmenopausal Women with Elevated Insulin Levels." *Nutr Res* 2009;29(11):768–76.

Kurz, A. "Physiology of Thermoregulation." *Baillieres Best Pract Res Clin Anaesthesiol* 2008;22(4):627–44.

Landsberg, L., J. B. Young, W. R. Leonard, R. A. Linsenmeier, and F. W. Turek. "Is Obesity Associated with Lower Body

Temperatures? Core Temperature: A Forgotten Variable in Energy Balance." *Metabolism* 2009;58(6):871–76.

Lemay, A., L. Turcot, F. Déchêne, S. Dodin, and J. C. Forest. "Hyperinsulinemia in Nonobese Women Reporting a Moderate Weight Gain at the Beginning of Menopause: A Useful Early Measure of Susceptibility to Insulin Resistance." *Menopause* 2010;17(2):321–25.

Lovejoy, J. C. "The Menopause and Obesity." *Prim Care* 2003;30(2): 317–25.

Manios, Y., G. Moschonis, K. Koutsikas, S. Papoutsou, I. Petraki, E. Bellou, A. Naoumi, S. Kostea, and S. Tanagra. "Changes in Body Composition Following a Dietary and Lifestyle Intervention Trial: The Postmenopausal Health Study." *Maturitas* 2009;62(1):58–65.

Marra, M., F. Pasanisi, C. Montagnese, E. De Filippo, C. De Caprio, L. de Magistris, and F. Contaldo. "BMR Variability in Women of Different Weight." *Clin Nutr* 2007;26(5):567–72.

McAndrew, L. M., M. A. Napolitano, A. Albrecht, N. C. Farrell, B. H. Marcus, and J. A. Whiteley. "When, Why and for Whom There Is a Relationship Between Physical Activity and Menopause Symptoms." *Maturitas* 2009;64(2):119–25.

Merchant, A. T., H. Vatanparast, S. Barlas, M. Dehghan, S. M. A. Shah, L. De Koning, and S. E. Steck. "Carbohydrate Intake and Overweight and Obesity among Healthy Adults." *J Am Diet Assoc* 2009;109(7):1165–72.

Metcalf, B. S., L. D. Voss, J. Hosking, A. N. Jeffery, and T. J. Wilkin. "Physical Activity at the Government-Recommended Level and Obesity-Related Health Outcomes: A Longitudinal Study." *Arch Dis Child* 2008;93(9):772–77.

Misso, M. L., C. Jang, J. Adams, J. Tran, Y. Murata, R. Bell, W. C. Boon, E. R. Simpson, and S. R. Davis. "Differential Expression of Factors Involved in Fat Metabolism with Age and the Menopause Transition." *Maturitas* 2005;51(3):299–306.

Miszko, T. A., and M. E. Cress. "A Lifetime of Fitness: Exercise in the Perimenopausal and Postmenopausal Woman." *Clin Sports Med* 2000;19(2):215–32.

Moran, L., and R. J. Norman. "Understanding and Managing Disturbances in Insulin Metabolism and Body Weight in Women with

Polycystic Ovary Syndrome." *Baillieres Best Pract Res Clin Obstet Gynaecol* 2004;18(5):719–36.

Nestares, T., L.-F. M. de la Higuera, J. Diaz-Castro, M. S. Campos, and M. López-Frías. "Evaluating the Effectiveness of a Weight-Loss Program for Perimenopausal Women." *Int J Vitam Nutr Res* 2009;79(4):212–17.

Nicklas, B. J., X. Wang, T. You, M. F. Lyles, J. Demons, L. Easter, M. J. Berry, L. Lenchik,and J. J. Carr. "Effect of Exercise Intensity on Abdominal Fat Loss during Calorie Restriction in Overweight and Obese Postmenopausal Women: A Randomized, Controlled Trial." *Am J Clin Nutr* 2009;89(4):1043–52.

Ohkawara, K., S. Tanaka, K. Ishikawa-Takata, and I. Tabata. "Twenty-Four-Hour Analysis of Elevated Energy Expenditure after Physical Activity in a Metabolic Chamber: Models of Daily Total Energy Expenditure." *Am J Clin Nutr* 2008;87(5):1268–76.

Parmar, H. S., and A. Kar. "Medicinal Values of Fruit Peels from *Citrus sinensis, Punica granatum,* and *Musa paradisiaca* with Respect to Alterations in Tissue Lipid Peroxidation and Serum Concentration of Glucose, Insulin, and Thyroid Hormones." *J Med Food* 2008;11(2):376–81.

Pasiakos, S. M., J. B. Mettel, K. West, I. E. Lofgren, M. L. Fernandez, S. I. Koo, and N. R. Rodriguez. "Maintenance of Resting Energy Expenditure after Weight Loss in Premenopausal Women: Potential Benefits of a High-Protein, Reduced-Calorie Diet." *Metabolism* 2008;57(4):458–64.

Pines, A. "Lifestyle and Diet in Postmenopausal Women. *Climacteric* 2009;12(Suppl 1):62–65.

Riesco, E., M. Roussel, S. Lemoine, S. Garnier, F. Sanguignol, and P. Mauriège. "What Is the Influence of Menopausal Status on Metabolic Profile, Eating Behaviors, and Perceived Health of Obese Women after Weight Reduction?" *Appl Physiol Nutr Metab* 2008;33(5):957–65.

Rumessen, J. J. "Fructose and Related Food Carbohydrates: Sources, Intake, Absorption, and Clinical Implications." *Scand J Gastroenterol* 1992;27(10):819–28.

Scott, C. B., and R. Devore. "Diet-Induced Thermogenesis: Variations among Three Isocaloric Meal-Replacement Shakes." *Nutrition* 2005;21(7):874–77.

Stewart, K. J., A. C. Bacher, P. S. Hees, M. Tayback, P. Ouyang, and S. Jan de Beur. "Exercise Effects on Bone Mineral Density: Relationships to Changes in Fitness and Fatness." *Am J Prev Med* 2005;28(5):453–60.

Steyer, T. E., and A. Ables. "Complementary and Alternative Therapies for Weight Loss." *Prim Care* 2009;36(2):395–406.

Tentolouris, N., C. Tsigos, D. Perea, E. Koukou, D. Kyriaki, E. Kitsou, S. Daskas, Z. Daifotis, K. Makrilakis, S. A. Raptis, and N. Katsilambros. "Differential Effects of High-Fat and High-Carbohydrate Isoenergetic Meals on Cardiac Autonomic Nervous System Activity in Lean and Obese Women." *Metabolism* 2003;52(11):1426–32.

Vicennati, V., F. Pasqui, C. Cavazza, U. Pagotto, and R. Pasquali. "Stress-Related Development of Obesity and Cortisol in Women." *Obesity (Silver Spring)* 2009;17(9):1678–83.

Wang, X., M. F. Lyles, T. You, M. J. Berry, W. J. Rejeski, and B. J. Nicklas. "Weight Regain Is Related to Decreases in Physical Activity during Weight Loss." *Med Sci Sports Exerc* 2008;40(10):1781–88.

Weinsier, R. L., K. M. Nelson, D. D. Hensrud, B. E. Darnell, G. R. Hunter, and Y. Schutz. "Metabolic Predictors of Obesity: Contribution of Resting Energy Expenditure, Thermic Effect of Food, and Fuel Utilization to Four-Year Weight Gain of Post-Obese and Never-Obese Women." *J Clin Invest* 1995;95(3):980–85.

Weltman, N. Y., S. A. Saliba, E. J. Barrett, and A. Weltman. "The Use of Exercise in the Management of Type 1 and Type 2 Diabetes." *Clin Sports Med* 2009;28(3):423–39.

Willett, W. C. "Dietary Fat and Body Fat: Is There a Relationship?" *J Nutr Biochem* 1998;9(9):522–24.

Winham, D. M., C. B. Collins, and A. M. Hutchins. "Dietary Intakes, Attitudes toward Carbohydrates of Postmenopausal Women Following Low Carbohydrate Diets." *Can J Diet Pract Res* 2009;70(1):44–47.

Yankura, D. J., M. B. Conroy, R. Hess, K. K. Pettee, L. H. Kuller, and A. M. Kriska. "Weight Regain and Health-Related Quality of Life in Postmenopausal Women." *Obesity (Silver Spring)* 2008;16(10):2259–65.

Zamboni, M., F. Armellini, E. Turcato, R. Micciolo, S. Desideri, I. A. Bergamo-Andreis, and O. Bosello. "Effect of Regain of Body Weight on Regional Body Fat Distribution: Comparison Between Pre- and Postmenopausal Obese Women." *Obes Res* 1996;4(6):555–60.

Zanesco, A., and P. R. Zaros. "Physical Exercise and Menopause." *Rev Bras Ginecol Obstet* 2009;31(5):254–61.

Zenk, J. L., S. A. Leikam, L. J. Kassen, and M. A. Kuskowski. "Effect of Lean System 7 on Metabolic Rate and Body Composition." *Nutrition* 2005;21(2):179–85.

Acknowledgments

If ever a book was more a process than a product, then this must be it.

Throughout the process many people contributed, in many consequential ways, to bringing the final product into being. Some individuals were especially imperative to the process and its success.

My partner, Ingrid, who stood by me through thick and thin, and who helped to keep the flame burning so this book would get to see the light of the day. No words can thank you enough.

My cowriter and friend, Robert Wolff, for believing that *Menopause Reset!* is more than just another diet book, who worked hard to turn my ideas into prose, and who contributed a writing perspective and expertise that will never be forgotten. His careful examinations of my text for language accuracy, clarity, and completeness and his ongoing efforts and feedback have been extraordinary and invaluable.

Shannon Welch and the great people at Rodale. Thank you for your passion, enthusiasm, and vision and for helping us create a book we are all so proud of.

Last but not least, Mel Berger and the William Morris Endeavor agency, who believed in and supported this book project from the beginning, for not giving up on me or on this book, and for ensuring that it became the best product possible. I am forever thankful.

Index